Religion and Sight

Religion and the Senses
Series Editor: Graham Harvey, The Open University, UK

Everyday and/or vernacular religions are now at the cutting edge of the study of religions. The agenda of Religious Studies as well as that of other disciplines which overlap in some aspects with the study of religion (e.g. Classics, History, Sociology, Anthropology and [in some places] Philosophy) has been revitalised by this focus on lived reality. This resonates with the growing interest in materiality and embodiment which have both provoked 'turns' in academic debate and teaching. Criticisms, however, have been levelled against the ways in which 'materiality' does not always engage with materials (stuff) and 'embodiment' sometimes suggests the priority of some interiority (mind, agency, etc.).

The proposed series aims to push further the project of placing lived, material and bodily religion at the definitive centre of studies of religion(s). It will do this by foregrounding bodily sensation and material practice as religion (rather than expressions, experiences or representations of something prior to bodies, acts and things). It develops the interdisciplinary conversation encouraged by Paul Stoller's *Sensuous Scholarship* (1997) and, especially, presents and promotes research about real life religion approached through performative and materialist methods, as illustrated by, e.g., Manuel Vasquez's *More than Belief* (2011) and Graham Harvey's *Food, Sex and Strangers* (2013).

Published:

Sensual Religion: Religion and the Five Senses
Edited by Graham Harvey and Jessica Hughes

Religion and Sight

Edited by
Louise Child and Aaron Rosen

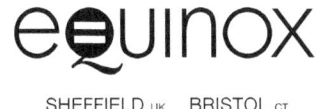

SHEFFIELD UK   BRISTOL CT

Published by Equinox Publishing Ltd.
UK: Office 415, The Workstation, 15 Paternoster Row, Sheffield, South Yorkshire S1 2BX
USA: ISD, 70 Enterprise Drive, Bristol, CT 06010

www.equinoxpub.com

First published 2020

© Louise Child, Aaron Rosen and contributors 2020

All rights reserved. No part of this publication may be reproduced or transmitted in any form or by any means, electronic or mechanical, including photocopying, recording or any information storage or retrieval system, without prior permission in writing from the publishers.

British Library Cataloguing-in-Publication Data
A catalogue record for this book is available from the British Library.

ISBN-13 978 1 78179 748 8 (hardback)
         978 1 78179 749 5 (paperback)
         978 1 78179 750 1 (ePDF)

Library of Congress Cataloging-in-Publication Data
Names: Child, Louise, 1966 - editor.
Title: Religion and sight / edited by Louise Child and Aaron Rosen.
Description: Bristol : Equinox Publishing Ltd, 2020. | Series: Religion and the senses | Includes bibliographical references and index. | Summary: 'Sight is both celebrated and denigrated in religion. In some contexts it is extolled as a source of knowledge and revelation. In others it is demonized as the road to illusion and idolatry. There is no single way that sight functions in religion, nor indeed a single way to study it. This edited volume brings together scholars from a wide range of disciplines - religious studies, anthropology, art history, film, and philosophy - to shed light on how the sense of sight shapes, and is shaped by, religion. Case studies range across both place and time, from narratives about Medusa in ancient Greek religion to spiritual explanations of sleepwalking in the Enlightenment to rituals of spirit possession in contemporary Brazil. In order to shed light on interconnected issues, the essays are grouped into three sections, moving thematically from darkness into light: 1) Obscurity 2) Altered States 3) Illumination. The contributors seek to avoid some of the historical pitfalls of Western discourses that hierarchize the senses, and in particular privilege and separate sight from the other senses, imagining it as an unimpeachable source of empirical knowledge. They present the ways in which sight transgresses such constructions, whether by being creatively misleading or taking on tactile qualities. Viewed in the context of lived religious experience, sight surfaces in multiple, unbounded ways. In a theoretically rich and self-reflective introduction, the volume editors set the stage by asking questions at the core of our discipline: What do we see, and-just as importantly-how do we see, when we study religion?' -- Provided by publisher.
Identifiers: LCCN 2019034185 (print) | LCCN 2019034186 (ebook) | ISBN 9781781797488 (hardback) | ISBN 9781781797495 (paperback) | ISBN 9781781797501 (ebook)
Subjects: LCSH: Revelation. | Vision--Religious aspects. | Religion.
Classification: LCC BL475.5 .R45 2020 (print) | LCC BL475.5 (ebook) | DDC 204/.2--dc23
LC record available at https://lccn.loc.gov/2019034185
LC ebook record available at https://lccn.loc.gov/2019034186

Typeset by S.J.I. Services, New Delhi, India

To Our Beloved Teachers

Graham Howes
and
Philip Mellor

Contents

List of Figures		ix
Series Foreword		xi
Graham Harvey		
Introduction: Setting Our Sights on Religion		1
Louise Child and Aaron Rosen		

Section One: Obscurity

1. Darkness Visible: The Art of Sam Winston 17
   Aaron Rosen

2. Visibly Invisible: Muslim Women in Twenty-first Century
   Political Cartoons 26
   Tahnia Ahmed

3. Obscuring Two-Spirit Deaths in the Films *Conversion* and *Fire Song* 46
   Gabriel Estrada

Section Two: Altered States

4. Sensing Reelism: Portals to Multiple Realities and Relationships
   in World, Indigenous and Documentary Cinema 69
   Louise Child

5 The Female Gaze: Sight and the Medusa Myth　　　　　　　　87
   Gina Bevan

6 'A Power Invisible': How Somnambulists' Blindness Reflected
   Debate on the Existence of the Soul　　　　　　　　　　　106
   Martina Bartlett

7 The Experience of Seeing: Spirit Possession as Performance　122
   Bettina E. Schmidt

Section Three: Illumination

8 Piet Mondrian's Abstraction as a Way of Seeing the Sacred　143
   Lieke Wijnia

9 Sacred Landscapes, New Conversations: Paul Nash's Visionary
   Paintings of the Wittenham Clumps　　　　　　　　　　　160
   Molly Kady

10 A Hand Outstretched in Darkness: Evangelical Encounters
   with Art　　　　　　　　　　　　　　　　　　　　　　182
   Philip Salim Francis

11 Seeing the Gods: Divine Embodiment through Visualisation in
   Tantric Buddhist Practice　　　　　　　　　　　　　　　200
   Dawn H. Collins

Index　　　　　　　　　　　　　　　　　　　　　　　　　221

List of Figures

1.1 Sam Winston, *Erasure of Blind Drawing*, 2016. Photo: Andy Sewell/Sam Winston. Courtesy of and © Sam Winston.   18

1.2 Sam Winston, *Blindfolded Text Drawing*, 2016. Photo: Andy Sewell/Sam Winston. Courtesy of and © Sam Winston.   20

1.3 Sam Winston, *Darkness Visible*, 2017, installation view, Southbank Centre, London. Photo: Pietro Martini. Courtesy of and © Sam Winston.   21

2.1 Mac, 'Doris, love. How would you like to feel empowered?' *Daily Mail*, 20 July 2010.   35

3.1 The respectful distance from death outside the hogan. *Conversion* (2006). Directed by Nanobah Becker. Park City, UT: Sundance Institute/Sundance Institute Native Initiative.   49

3.2 David holds Shane by the rice fields. *Fire Song* (2015). Directed by Adam Garnet Jones. Toronto: Big Soul Productions.   60

7.1 Ceremony in the Yoruba-Orisha Baptist Church in Brooklyn, New York City. Photo by Bettina E. Schmidt, 15 February 1998.   125

7.2 Caribbean Carnival parade in Brooklyn, New York City. Photo by Bettina E. Schmidt, 6 September 1999.   128

7.3 Candomblé ceremony in São Paulo. Photo by Bettina E. Schmidt, 24 April 2010.   132

7.4 Umbanda ceremony in São Paulo. Photo by Bettina E. Schmidt, 11 April 2010.   136

9.1 The Wittenham Clumps, December, 2017. Photo by Graham
    Harvey. © Molly Kady. 161
9.2 John and Paul Nash, *Poster Design*, 1913. Private collection of
    Ms Anne Drew. 168
9.3 Paul Nash, *The Wood on the Hill*, 1912. © Ashmolean Museum,
    University of Oxford. 174
9.4 Paul Nash, *Landscape of the Summer Solstice*, 1943. National
    Gallery of Victoria, Melbourne. 177
11.1 A Tibetan silk painting (T. *thang kha*) depicting the divine realm
    (S. *maṇḍala*) of the Medicine Buddha. Photo by Dawn H. Collins. 203
11.2 Rebgong spirit-medium (*lawa*) at the Leru. Photo by
    Dawn H. Collins. 205
11.3 Tantric practitioners in Rebgong. Photo by Dawn H. Collins. 207
11.4 Palden Lhamo statue in a Rebgong temple for the local deities.
    Photo by Dawn H. Collins. 211
11.5 Lhamolhatso Lake. Photo by Dawn H. Collins. 212
11.6 Shurwu Tongdok ritual offerings. Photo by Dawn H. Collins. 215
11.7 A *thang kha* depicting Palden Lhamo with retinue, Chötsen
    Donchen to her right and Sengé Donchen to her left.
    Charitable Assistance Society, Phuntsok Cho Ling Buddhist
    Centre, public domain. 217

Series Foreword

GRAHAM HARVEY

Religion is sensual because it is corporeal and earthy. Religion is something that people (always bodies) do in the world (always physical). It is seen, heard, tasted, smelled and touched and often involves senses of place, decency, awe, humour, value and honour. These and other senses work together (although not always successfully), and they are integral to corporeality and to engagement with the world. Some of our experiences privilege particular senses—as when we close our eyes to better appreciate music. The sensual impact of religious activities can be staged to employ or heighten one sense at a time, perhaps allowing incense or singing to take a lead. Or they can work together as when the burning of incense coincides with the ringing of bells to direct attention. There are myriad ramifications. This series engages with a wide range of such matters.

It is true that some religions make the physical senses a battleground: encouraging the suppression of bodily senses and desires in favour of 'more spiritual' leanings. In doing so, they do not contradict the assertion that religion is sensual but, rather, they evidence it. Progress in seeking putatively non-material gains or experiences, or of seeking mystical and transcendent states, may be recognised by degrees of success in restraining the more everyday senses. If these senses are not restrained, they may be trained to serve "more elevated" purposes. Paying attention to the feeling of inward and outward breathing to initiate mindfulness does not negate sensuality but employs it. The banning of music creates alternative sonic environments (e.g. of silence or spoken words) that are deemed suitable to the feel of some ways of being religious. Similarly, quasi-cyborg interactions in online and virtual religion do not challenge the sensuality of religious activities but are conducted through the touch of keyboards, sight of screens and hearing of digital sounds. Examples could be multiplied.

This series has deep foundations in approaches to religion which emphasise the everyday, practice or performance, materiality, embodiment and affect. It owes much to the scholarship of religion and gender which brings into sharp focus the importance of attending to lived realities and refuses to waft away the stench of patriarchal power dynamics. *Religion and the Senses* begins with the assumption that religion is something people do. For some people, this 'doing of religion' is especially about cognition: the encouragement of correct believing or correct understanding. These activities have been emphasised by scholars as well as religious practitioners in most publications about religion. However, religion is as much about the preparation, eating and waste-management of the foods people eat or avoid as it is about the putative meanings of food-rules. Communities are made by eating together, sharing appropriate foods at appropriate times, and equally by avoiding inappropriate foods and those who eat them. They may be riven by the wearing of the wrong costume or by visual or auditory attention to inappropriate media. Religious conflicts can be less about differences of belief than about the censorial setting apart of sensory worlds.

Religion and the Senses builds on these relatively familiar perspectives on lived religion. However, the series is more than summative of existing knowledge. It seeks to advance the cutting edge of debates. It is provocative because it engages with the sensuality of religion on the understanding that religion is *fully* sensual, corporeal and earthy. It pushes further an existing project in which religious senses largely serve to enhance appreciation of the lived reality of religions. Great advances in understanding and analysing religion have been made. However, just as debates about 'materiality' have not always engaged with materials (stuff) and those about 'embodiment' have sometimes suggested the priority of some interiority (mind, agency, etc.), so those about religion and the senses have sometimes suggested that 'religion' exists before and apart from senses. In the books which comprise *Religion and the Senses*, religion will be pursued as something that is not merely represented by or expressed in sensual data (e.g. arts and acts), but is a matter of bodies moving through the world. Attending to sensuality does not (merely) add colour and drama to our views of religion(s). It is not only about the vignettes that introduce our debates. Religion is the smelling, tasting, touching, hearing and seeing of the world in particular ways. We need to attend to everything from bodily affects to trained enculturation (not to evoke a nature/culture dualism but to indicate a rich diversity of topics) in order to understand how sensual religion propels people in their daily and ritual negotiations with life.

This foreword has made use of the conventional idea that there are five senses, albeit with some recognition that these can or must work together (sometimes conflictually). However, the series is not restricted to discussion of those five senses or their synaesthetic interactions. These are our entry points, our 'starting from where we are' places. The journey towards a richer and fuller sense of religion will entail a much wider notion of senses. It will require us to explore senses of place, decorum, decency, value, health/well-being, the uncanny, humour, honour and others. These 'extra' senses provide even greater possibilities for considering movement, relationships, interactions, locations and other matters.

Some of these 'senses' might make more immediate sense than others—e.g. sense of place is a relatively familiar theme in discussing religious locations and commitments. Sense of value encourages consideration of religion and economic systems (e.g. capitalist, gift, votive and sacrificial economies), charity or philanthropy, and of ultimate versus putatively lesser 'needs' or concerns. Sense of decorum might bring discussions of religion and costume into dialogue with discussions of religious discipline and deportment (e.g. stipulations that elders should not run, children should be silent, women should be humble). Sense of honour can generate acts of violence against perceived wrong-doers as well as celebration of specific practices. The sense of the uncanny brings us face-to-face with the worlds of possession and ghosts, with feelings of unease or dread that may require the employment of religious specialists. In contrast with sense of place perhaps the sense of the uncanny is about dislocation and un-ease in the presence of the unknown, unexpected or unwelcome. As these presences are sometimes faced with edgy trickster tales, they provide an additional reason (if we needed it) to immerse ourselves in the sense of humour. If nothing else, jokes told within a religion (about that religion or about others) are revelatory of what is truly at the heart of that lifeway. Reiterating the synaesthetic and corporeal nature of all the senses, perhaps these religious jokes sometimes provoke throaty chortles or 'belly laughs'. Engaging with these many and varied, but usually interacting senses will require authors and readers to confront a broad spectrum of religious acts and ideas, some more edgy or contested than others.

There are, in short, many good reasons for studying religion and the senses, including the assertion made by this foreword (and contested both by some religionists and by perhaps within some of the following chapters) that religion is fully and definitively sensual, corporeal and worldly. This series takes up the project of the 'turns' to lived religion, everyday religion, materiality, gender, embodiment and performance. By sustained focus on the senses—perhaps mediating mechanisms between our bodies and our world—we will gain a greatly improved sense of what religion is and what religious people do.

Dr Graham Harvey is professor of religious studies at The Open University. His research interests contribute to his broader, long-term engagement with material- and lived-religion; his recent research largely concerns "the new animism," especially in the rituals and protocols through which Indigenous and other communities engage with the larger-than-human world. Harvey's publications include *Food, Sex and Strangers: Understanding Religion as Everyday Life* (2013) and *Animism: Respecting the Living World* (2nd edition 2017). He is editor of the Equinox series *Religion and the Senses*, the first volume of which, *Sensual Religion: Religion and the Five Senses* (2018), he co-edited with Jessica Hughes. He is also the editor of *Indigenising in European Religious Movements* (2020).

Introduction: Setting Our Sights on Religion

LOUISE CHILD AND AARON ROSEN

Human egotism—what some ethicists refer to as speciesism—often leads us to be a bit too proud of our senses. We celebrate the palette of a chef, the nose of a parfumier, the dexterity of an athlete, and the eyesight of a pilot. Yet the truth is that there is no single sense that humans possess that is not more acute in another creature on earth.

When it comes to sight, we not only lack the razor-sharp acuity of birds of prey but even the nocturnal vision of the average housecat. Still, for a species with relatively underwhelming achievements in other senses, it is understandable that we often place a high value on vision. Whether we are spotting predators, foraging for grub, or building relationships by looking at one another, sight has been formative in our evolution. We can do without sight—and of course some have done so ingeniously—but it is, literally, hardwired into the human brain in complex, important ways, some of which we are only just beginning to understand scientifically.

Vision is not simply the reception of a dataset but the staggeringly complicated collating and interpretation of information. This is brought out memorably in the titular story of neurologist Oliver Sacks' book *The Man Who Mistook His Wife for a Hat*. Sacks narrates the case of a patient with visual agnosia, a condition characterised by an incapacity to recognise familiar objects, or even people, despite 'seeing' them clearly. The ability to see clearly might feel instantaneous, intuitive, even quotidian, but it is—biologically speaking—miraculous.

SEEING IS BELIEVING?

This brings us to the topic of our book: religion and sight. Many religions have claimed literally miraculous powers for sight, often predicated upon a limited knowledge of biology. In Jewish and Christian tradition, sight begins with God, unseen yet all-seeing, disembodied yet perceiving. According to Genesis, 'the earth was a formless void and darkness covered the face of the deep.... Then God said, "Let there be light"; and there was light. And God saw that the light was good' (Gen. 1.2–4). By this account, God not only creates the conditions for visual perception by dividing light from dark, God participates in this sensory act before doing anything else. Not only is light 'good,' sight is too.

How different would Western religious and philosophical discourse have been, we might wonder, if the Hebrew Bible had pictured God touching light, or smelling the earth before declaring it pleasing? Even for God, it seems, seeing is believing. Sight, of all possible modes of apprehension—intellectual or sensorial—makes creation comprehensible, makes it *real*. As the Bible progresses, and it is humanity's turn to look, confirm and pronounce things good, sight continues to exert a validating force. As the Israelites make the long, arduous journey from Egypt to the Promised Land, Moses prevails upon them to hold fast to their God, 'who has done for you these great and awesome things that your own eyes have seen' (Deut. 10.21). Recognising the Israelites' tendency to go astray, Moses does not challenge the people to professions of blind faith. Instead, he reminds them that they have witnessed with their 'own eyes' everything they need to know to follow God.

In the New Testament, sight might appear, on first reading, to take a backseat to belief. When Jesus first appears to his disciples after his resurrection, one follower, Thomas, is absent. Thomas refuses to take the others' testimony at face value, insisting he will not believe Jesus has returned from the dead unless he is able to cast his own eyes upon his master's pierced flesh. When Thomas finally beholds Jesus, his teacher gently reproves him: 'Have you believed because you have seen me? Blessed are those who have not seen and yet have come to believe' (John 20.29). Physical sight is not so much downgraded here as displaced. We should not need to see, the passage implies, because others have seen before us, *for us*. At the same time that John critiques Thomas' reliance on sight, he encourages us to benefit from Thomas' incredulity. If the dubious disciple was convinced on the spot by what he witnessed, surely we have all the evidence we need. Ironically, a story which seems to elevate faith above sight depends upon the veracity of vision.

In its early centuries, as Christianity sought to affirm its truth claims over and against its rivals, Christian thinkers accused Jews of ignoring the evidence right in front of their (or their ancestors') faces: Jesus was the Messiah their own scriptures foretold. Saint Augustine diagnosed them with 'nearsightedness' (p. 171), explaining:

> The Jews'd retain as their own, if nothing else of their Divine Inheritance, only the Divine Scripture. Why this harsh Justice? Alas, they'd closed their eyes to the meaning of Scripture. In it the Jews'd continue to carry the proof of Salvation, but not for them. For us! Yes, these were the very same writings that'd open the eyes of the Gentiles. (p. 172)

In the middle ages, the trope of the blind Jew and the prescient gentile crystallised in the popular iconography of *synagoga* and *ecclesia*, the synagogue and the church, embodied by contrasting female figures, often sculpted on cathedral facades. The slumped *synagoga* appeared with blindfolded or downcast eyes, clasping the tablets of the law, whilst *ecclesia* held a chalice and cross and looked confidently ahead. Vision, it seems, had become a hereditary affair, with Jews destined to inherit the myopia of their ancestors, and Christians the acuity of their forebears. Where early followers of Christ had emphasised that seeing is believing—making claims based on 'eyewitnesses' (Luke 1.2; cf. John 20.8, 20.31)—as Christianity developed it came to view sight as a spiritual faculty. If seeing is believing, believing can also be a type of seeing.

The notion that 'believing is seeing' is not simply metaphorical, nor is it exclusive to Christianity, as Dawn Collins and other authors in this volume demonstrate. Numerous religions describe mystical encounters with the divine in effulgent terms, at times giving specific instructions—whether via incantation, meditation, deprivation, intoxication or other ritual acts— for practitioners to achieve illumination. At the centre of many such experiences is a 'hierophany,' defined by the phenomenologist Mircea Eliade as 'the manifestation of something of a wholly different order, a reality that does not belong to our world' (1959: 11). These experiences might run the gamut from solitary 'vision quests' undertaken in pursuit of sacred objects or animals by indigenous peoples in North America to mind-blowing theophanies, in which the nature of the universe itself is disclosed. In the *Bhagavad Gita*, the warrior Arjuna entreats the Hindu god Krishna to reveal himself in his universal form. Krishna responds 'you cannot see Me with your present eyes. Therefore I give to you divine eyes by which you can behold My mystic opulence' (11.8). Safely protected by these 'divine eyes,' as if preparing to witness a solar eclipse, Arjuna beholds a retina-searing spectacle. 'If hundreds of thousands of suns rose up at once into the sky,' we are told, 'they might resemble the effulgence of the Supreme Person in that universal form' (11.12). In a Greek myth retold by Ovid, the woman Semele persuades her lover Zeus, against his better judgement, to show himself in his true form. Unable to withstand his splendour, she dies instantly. Ken Dowden explains that 'Zeus is an unseen force of incalculable power. Only Semele seeks to see that power as it really is and her mortal frame cannot withstand the thunderbolt that *is* Zeus' (2006: 48).[1] Attempting to apprehend divine reality with human vision—especially for the uninitiated or ritually unprepared—can be a fatal category mistake.

Hindu and Greek mythology use poetic language to paint dazzling pictures of sensory overload. Yet visual artists have often attempted to capture something of the sublime directly, whether in traditional media like paint or stained glass, or new media such as digital projections. In the medieval period, for instance, one might think of the words Abbot Suger inscribed on the doors of Saint-Denis in Paris. Its revolutionary stained-glass windows, he hoped, would 'brighten the minds, so that they may travel, through the true lights | To the True Light ...' (Frisch 1987: 7). Muslim architects and artisans likewise sought to create works that would transport viewers from the earthly to heavenly realm. One might think of the ornate geometry of the Alhambra complex in Granada, Spain, from the constellated ceiling symbolising the seven heavens in the Hall of the Ambassadors to the muqarnas vaulting of the Dome of the Two Sisters (both of the fourteenth century), in which the contemporary Iberian poet Ibn Zamrak found intimations of eternity (Hillenbrand 1998: 195).

If looking at art constitutes one way to channel the divine, creating it can be another conduit. Orhan Pamuk, in *My Name is Red*, describes how master manuscript illuminators in the Ottoman Empire longed to become blind in old age as a reward for their scrupulosity, drawing them away from the realm of physical to transcendental beauty. Here physical and spiritual sight seem to exist on a continuum, with one sharpening as the other fades. In the present volume, several chapters reflect on the ways in which modern artists have sought to unlock a form of supra-sensory spiritual

---

1 Other examples include complex treatises about vision, visions and the sight of God in Judaism in which there are suggestions that the sight of God can cause sudden death (Wolfson 1994: e.g. 362, 133).

perception by visual means. Lieke Wijnia sheds new light on the Dutch abstract painter Piet Mondrian, who felt he was entering such uncharted territory in his radical compositions that he needed to coin new words to describe the visionary experience he wanted viewers to have. Molly Kady examines another avant-garde painter, the English surrealist Paul Nash, who came to regard the Oxfordshire landscape through an animist lens, sensing that it contained a mythic, regenerative power. Philip Francis, in this book's penultimate chapter, explores how experiencing works of modern and contemporary art might 'facilitate the process by which [American evangelicals] literally *see and feel* their way out of evangelicalism and into other social units.' Looking at art, as Francis demonstrates, can catalyse an alternative act—or indeed art—of self-formation.

TOUCHING SIGHT

It is difficult, if not downright impossible, to disentangle sight from the other senses. Whilst Western religious and philosophical traditions have tended to elevate and separate sight from the other senses—seeking to preserve its ostensibly rational, empirical character—artists and writers have often intuitively known better.[2] In the early twentieth century, Wassily Kandinsky penned a short treatise *Concerning the Spiritual in Art*, in which he posited that the integration of sight with the other senses was crucial in order for visual art to reach its spiritual potential. He wrote:

> [C]olour is a power which directly influences the soul. Colour is the keyboard, the eyes are the hammers, the soul is the piano with many strings. The artist is the hand which plays, touching one key or another, to cause vibrations in the soul. (Kandinsky 1977: 25)

Inspired by his own cognitive condition of synaesthesia, which meant that he experienced colours as sounds as well as sights, Kandinsky sought to create holistic experiences for viewers, whom he hoped would *listen* to paintings he titled 'Fugues,' 'Compositions' and 'Improvisations.'[3] George Eliot, writing with inimitable sensitivity, recognised that the ability to truly sense the world around us—and especially the presence of others—might

---

2 Martin Jay helpfully identifies a counter-tradition in *Downcast Eyes: The Denigration of Vision in Twentieth-Century French Thought* (1993).
3 Pamuk, mentioned above, posits similarly: 'Colour is the touch of the eye, music to the deaf, a word out of the darkness.'

not only prove revelatory but immobilising. 'If we had a keen vision and feeling of all ordinary human life,' she writes, 'it would be like hearing the grass grow and the squirrel's heart beat, and we should die of that roar which lies on the other side of silence' (1994: 194). In our own volume, the artist Sam Winston speaks to Aaron Rosen about his experience creating works in total darkness as well as inviting audiences into immersive dark spaces. 'For me,' he reflects, 'it's about exploring this liminal transition between one sensory form and another, between sight and touch, or sight and sound. It's about trying to cope using different strategies in a completely different landscape....' He notes how sustained periods of sight deprivation can induce unusual perceptual experiences, difficult to assign to traditional sensory categories, not unlike the hypnagogic states studied by Martina Bartlett in her chapter.

As Winston's visual experiments suggest, touch not only augments sight, it can constitute a *form* of seeing, and vice versa. Émile Durkheim raises this possibility almost as an aside in his elaboration of the division between the sacred and the profane among aboriginal peoples in Australia.[4] When discussing prohibitions regarding sacred entities, he writes:

> [C]ontact can be established by means other than touching. One is in contact with a thing simply by looking at it; the gaze is a means of establishing contact. This is why, in certain cases, the sight of certain things is forbidden to the profane. A woman must never see the cult instruments and at most is allowed to glimpse them from afar...a corpse, too, is sometimes taken out of sight, the face being covered in such a way that it cannot be seen. (Durkheim 1995 [1912]: 308)

Diana Eck explores the continuum between sight and touch in Hindu worship. The central act of *darśan*, she explains, is a two-way process between divine beings—embodied by sacred figures or images—and devotees. '[T]he gaze of the huge eyes of the image meets that of the worshipper, and that exchange of vision lies at the heart of Hindu worship' (Eck 1985 [1981]: 7). Therefore, she argues, 'in the Indian context, seeing is a kind of touching', as well as a transmission of knowledge (p. 9). In many

---

4 It is important to be aware of key critical engagements with Durkheim's theories by modern anthropologists who have deeper engagements with indigenous traditions. His insistence on sharp divides between the sacred and the profane, for example, is thought to be overdrawn and misleading in many cases because indigenous traditions often emphasise the importance of all life, and religion can be found in many everyday activities of human and non-human persons (Harvey 2013).

ways, it is only from the later part of the twentieth century onwards that Western philosophical accounts of the senses—led by Maurice Merleau-Ponty—have begun to recognise the haptic dimensions of sight, which have long been part of many practitioners' lived religious experiences.

In this volume, Gina Bevan analyses the ancient Greek myth of Medusa, an example *par excellence* of the imbrication of sight and touch. As Bevan demonstrates, the idea of the gorgon's gaze—which exerted a deathly grip on viewers—reveals gendered discourses about who should wield the privilege of vision, and when. Questions about control and manipulation of the female gaze also surface in Tahnia Ahmed's chapter, in which she examines how Muslim women have been depicted in recent British political cartoons. She finds that images of veiled women often figure them as functionally invisible, and thus culturally and politically suspicious or subversive. On the other hand, they are also frequently depicted as victims of Muslim male control, in need of 'liberating' by enlightened Westerners. Gabriel Estrada calls our attention to another postcolonial context, and another medium, in which vision is implicated in a complex interplay between gender, sexuality, ethnicity and religion. Ze sensitively unpacks how recent films have obscured the deaths of lesbian, gay, bisexual, transgender and queer Indigenous people, who are at high risk of abuse, violence and suicide. Sight is not only a sense, it is a tool, and it can be deployed with equal efficacy to reveal, distort or conceal the machinations of power.

VISION PROBLEMS

We are acutely aware in assembling this volume that a focus on sight can be rewarding but also problematic. After all, the recent revolution in academic thinking about the senses has been driven, in large part, by a desire to move away from sight, or to situate it alongside other senses. For example, in *Aroma: The Cultural History of Smell*, Constance Classen, David Howes and Anthony Synott seek to recover a seat at the table for senses such as smell and taste, which have long been ignored. They write:

> The devaluation of smell in the contemporary west is directly linked to the revaluation of the senses which took place during the eighteenth and nineteenth centuries. The philosophers and scientists of that period decided that while sight was the pre-eminent sense of reason and civilization, smell was the sense of madness and savagery. In the course of human evolution, it was argued by Darwin, Freud and others, the sense of smell had been left behind and that of sight had taken priority. (1994: 3-4)

Rethinking such hierarchies has profound implications not only for the writing of intellectual and cultural history, but also for conducting fieldwork. Anthropology emerged as a discipline in the late nineteenth century, at a time when the sensory hierarchies noted above had largely solidified. Reorienting scholarship on the senses thus also means learning to conduct fieldwork in ways which do not simply reinforce or recapitulate sensory hierarchies but are open to alternative configurations.

Paul Stoller argues convincingly for the need for scholars to develop an attentiveness to alternative models of perception. His own lengthy immersion and repeated visits to communities in Niger opened up his sensory receptivity, and in turn broadened his approach to ethnography. He reflects:

> I let the sights, sounds, smells, and tastes of Niger flow into me. This fundamental rule in epistemological humility taught me that taste, smell, and hearing are often more important for the Songhay than sight, the privileged sense of the West. In Songhay one can taste kinship, smell witches, and hear the ancestors. (1989: 5)

This 'epistemological humility' can be just as hard to adopt when it comes to studying sensory experiences in Western religious communities, which scholars often expect to hew to established hierarchies. Robert Orsi's now classic cultural history of Italian Harlem in New York City, published in 1985, challenged conventions about what 'counts' as religious studies with its treatment of festivals and other embodied practices. Reflecting back on this work in 2002, Orsi notes how he came to understand that even the category of 'popular religion,' ostensibly meant to encompass the embodied realities of everyday religious experience, was really 'a code for Catholic-like ritual and devotional practices, deemed inappropriate and even incomprehensible on the religious landscape of the United States' (2002: xvii). In other words, how scholars look at religion—or indeed religious looking itself—is often influenced by religious optics; in this case a Protestant aversion to overtly sensual material.

Cultural frameworks of perception can be so naturalised that they can directly influence how scholars see what is right in front of them, even dictating their observations of basic characteristics such as size, shape and colour. C. Roderick Wilson, for example, reports not 'seeing' the purple hue of leaves on a distant Amazonian hilltop in the same way as his informants did. His habitual assumption that leaves are green had 'blinded' him to the purple effect of viewing the tree-covered hillsides from the vantage point of the village (2012 [1984]: 198–199).⁵ Within a religious context, a number of ethnographers have reported expanded or enhanced senses of sight whilst experiencing rituals. Edith Turner describes seeing a spirit during an African healing ritual (2006: 43). In this volume, Bettina Schmidt reports seeing individuals seem to take on different heights and other characteristics—for example appearing older and infirm—in the context of an Umbanda possession ceremony in Brazil. As Schmidt discusses, whilst such perceptions might have been considered too subjective by previous generations of anthropologists, today scholars are finding new ways to incorporate their visual and other sensory experiences into their analysis of rituals. Jean-Guy Goulet presses even further, suggesting the value of proffering one's own dreams and visions, both to informants and academic audiences. He argues that this level of immersion in the life-worlds of those one studies engenders trust, elicits information, and provides important material that derives from the penetration of the self by the host culture (2012 [1994]: 16–20). For her part, Louise Child in this volume considers whether the arts and non-documentary films might sometimes offer the best possible medium by which to capture experiential dynamics that evade an anthropologist's documentary lens or notepad.

These sightings suggest that a deeper sensorial engagement with the life-worlds of cultures under study implies a penetration of the observer, who is in some way—whether large or small—changed by the encounter. On one level, this indicates the need to identify, and in many cases revise, one's own preconceptions and cultural frameworks. On another level, it invites an opening up of dialogue about one's own sensual life. In some cases, this might involve acknowledging how the content of one's dreams, or even waking experiences, could be affected by the entrance of human, ancestral and spirit persons. Stoller, for instance, suggests that an experience of sleep paralysis, and his ability to ward off the symptoms by reciting a spell, was not only an indication of someone's ability to exercise power over him, but was also a precursor to being initiated into a higher level of training in sorcery. Complex ethical and methodological questions about

---

5   Scholars across the humanities and sciences, meanwhile, have long puzzled over Homer's repeated description of the 'wine-dark sea' in the *Iliad* and the *Odyssey*. Explanations have ranged from suggestions that the ancient Greeks suffered congenital colour-blindness, to the notion that minerals led to blue-tinted wine, or that algae regularly rendered the Aegean seas red (Wilford 1983: C1). Of course the most likely explanation remains that the Greeks simply enjoyed a different cultural vantage point, and chose poetic language accordingly.

sensual scholarship are also raised by several papers in the edited collection *Taboo: Sex, Identity and Erotic Subjectivity in Anthropological Fieldwork* (Kulick and Wilson 1995). For example, some scholars' use of metaphors of penetration and sensual seduction to explain and justify their participatory stance as observers in a community evoke troubling parallels with colonial engagements with colonised peoples. A great deal of work remains to be done about the best ways to navigate such spaces with ethical as well as perceptual sensitivity.

When anthropologists undergo initiations with religious groups, additional questions emerge about sensual scholarship. Initiated members of a religious group, for example, may see and touch religious images and other objects that are otherwise forbidden to non-initiates. André Singer's film *Fieldwork: Sir Walter Baldwin Spencer 1860–1929* (1986) broaches the issue of different understandings of such privileges and obligations from the perspectives of both anthropologists and the societies they study. The film explains that Spencer and his colleague Francis James Gillen removed sacred objects from Australian aboriginal tribes, including the Aranda (also spelt Arunta), and used these objects for public, national and international educational purposes such as museum collections. Although Gillen was granted initiation by the tribe, the film suggests that the Aranda could not have imagined, let alone understood, the implications of giving him permission to see their sacred objects.

Recent exhibitions have sought to be sensitive to these dilemmas when displaying creations by native peoples. For the British Museum's flagship exhibition *Indigenous Australia: Enduring Civilisation* (23 April–2 August 2015) curators sought permissions from the descendants of the original owners of objects before placing them on display. A number of objects were withheld or partly covered, and pixelated in catalogue reproductions, in order to prevent non-native audiences from viewing sacred or otherwise sensitive objects (Singh 2015). In some cases, indigenous peoples noted that this was actually for the protection of Western viewers themselves, for whom they believed the sight of powerful sacred works could prove physically harmful (Singh 2015). Visitors were prohibited from taking photographs, and images on postcards were carefully circumscribed, in order to prevent objects from being viewed in contexts of which elders did not approve (Singh 2015). Related questions come into play when visual materials produced for religious purposes by aboriginal peoples become inspiration for, or are directly sold as, art in the global market. As Howard Morphy points out, aboriginal peoples have in some cases developed intricate artistic strategies of concealing and revealing (1991). Techniques such as dot painting protect a principle of secrecy whilst producing work that can be appreciated aesthetically by outsiders, allowing creators to participate in some of the cultural and material benefits of art production in the contemporary global context.

Studying the power and efficacy—even unto death—of aboriginal creations within traditional networks of meaning and social relations can helpfully steer us towards productive questions that are often ignored within art history. In his final book, *Art and Agency: An Anthropological Theory*, Alfred Gell uses a wide range of examples drawn from Oceania to argue for a study of visual creations which deal seriously with how they operate as forms of 'social technology' (1998: 74). As he points out, 'the distinction we make between "mere" decoration and function is unwarranted; decoration is intrinsically functional' (1998: 74). W. J. T. Mitchell draws out related questions of agency in his memorably titled book, *What Do Pictures Want?* Discussing a plethora of subjects, from contemporary sculpture to film, advertising and biocybernetic reproductions, Mitchell sets out 'to look at the peculiar tendency of images to absorb and be absorbed by human subjects in processes that look suspiciously like those of living things' (2005: 2). Rather than regressing toward the 'primitive,' engaging with these anthropomorphic dimensions has the potential to free up deeper understandings of what art really does, especially in religious contexts. Indeed, one advantage may ultimately be to free scholars from some of the strictures and baggage implied by the term 'art,' which at times does more to stymie lines of inquiry than open them. A number of scholars are pursuing fruitful work in this liminal territory. Among others, we might think of: David Morgan on mass-produced religious imagery (1999); Kathryn Lofton on celebrity (2017); S. Brent Plate on stones and bread (2014); Sally Promey on Hawai'i Volcanoes National Park (2014); Jamal Elias on Pakistani truck painting (2011); and Birgit Meyer on Ghanaian videos (2015). A less blinkered approach to both religion and sight promises investigations in other, as yet uncharted areas.

Surveying such diverse possibilities for the study of religion and sight, taking place across multiple disciplines, is a daunting prospect. We have ultimately opted in this volume to favour inquiries that do not so much look to a distant future for the field as attempt to give a clear picture of where it stands now, right before our eyes. These close examinations invariably mean that a number of important subjects will be relegated to the reader's peripheral vision. At the same time, we hope that these eleven chapters will suggest numerous avenues for further inquiries into religion and sight, and indeed open the door for the coming volumes in this series on *Religion and the Senses*. After problematising visual metaphors like enlightenment in this introduction, we hope readers will pardon us the decision to organise this book into three sections which summon a rather teleological sense of progress, from Obscurity to Altered States to Illumination. Readers should of course feel more than welcome to read this book backwards, or indeed any way they want. After all, perhaps nothing is more religiously significant than to be left in a state of profound darkness.

FILM

Singer, André. (1986) *Fieldwork: Sir Walter Baldwin Spencer (1860-1929)*. UK: Central Independent Television.

BIBLIOGRAPHY

Augustine of Hippo. (2002) 'Sermo CC: Epiphany #2,' *Sermons to the People: Advent, Christmas, New Year's Epiphany*, translated and edited by William Griffin. New York: Doubleday, pp. 169–175.

Brehrend, H., Dreschke, A. and Zillinger, M. (eds.) (2014) *Trance Mediums and New Media: Spirit Possession in the Age of Technical Reproduction*. New York: Fordham University Press.

Classen, C., Howes, D. and Synott, A. (1994) *Aroma: The Cultural History of Smell*. London and New York: Routlege.

Dowden, Ken. (2006) *Zeus*. London and New York: Routledge.

Dundes, A. (ed.) (1981) *The Evil Eye: A Casebook*. New York and London: Garland.

Durkheim, Émile. (1995 [1912]) *The Elementary Forms of Religious Life* (translated from the French by Karen E. Fields). New York and London: The Free Press.

Eck, Diana. (1985 [1981]) *Darśan: Seeing the Divine Image in India*. Chamsbersberg, PA: Anima Books.

Eliade, Mircea. (1959) *The Sacred and the Profane: The Nature of Religion* (translated by Willard Trask). Orlando, FL: Harcourt.

Elias Jamal. (2011) *On Wings of Diesel: Trucks, Identity and Culture in Pakistan*. Oxford: Oneworld.

Elias, Jamal. (2012) *Aisha's Cushion: Religious Art, Perception, and Practice in Islam*. Cambridge, MA: Harvard University Press.

Eliot, George. (1994) *Middlemarch*. London: Penguin.

Frisch, Teresa. (ed.). (1987) *Gothic Art 1140-c. 1450: Sources and Documents*. Toronto: University of Toronto Press.

Gell, Alfred. (1998) *Art and Agency: An Anthropological Theory*. Oxford: Oxford University Press.

Geurts, K. L. (2003) 'On Embodied Consciousness in Anlo-Ewe Worlds: A Cultural Phenomenology of the Fetal Position,' *Ethnography* 4(3), 363–395.

Goulet, Jean-Guy. (2012 [1994]) 'Dreams and Other Lifeworlds,' in Young, D. E. and Goulet, J. (eds.), *Being Changed by Cross-Cultural Encounters: The Anthropology of Extraordinary Experience*. Ontario: University of Toronto Press, pp. 16–38.
Harvey, Graham. (2013) *Food, Sex and Strangers: Understanding Religion as Everyday Life*. Durham: Acumen.
Harvey, Graham and Hughes, J. (2018) *Sensual Religion: Religion and the Five Senses*. Sheffield and Bristol: Equinox.
Hillenbrand, Robert. (1998). *Islamic Art and Architecture*. London: Thames & Hudson.
Howes, D. (ed.) (2005) *Empire of the Senses: The Sensual Culture Reader*. Oxford and New York: Berg.
Howes, D. and Classen, C. (2013) *Ways of Sensing: Understanding the Senses in Society*. New York: Routledge.
Jay, Martin. (1993) *Downcast Eyes: The Denigration of Vision in Twentieth-Century French Thought*. Berkeley, CA: University of California Press.
Kandinsky, Wassily. (1977) *Concerning the Spiritual in Art* (translated by M. T. H. Sadler). New York: Dover.
Kulick, D. and Wilson, M. (eds.) (1995) *Taboo: Sex, Identity and Erotic Subjectivity in Anthropo-logical Fieldwork*. London and New York: Routledge.
Lofton, Kathryn. (2017) *Consuming Religion*. Chicago: University of Chicago Press.
Merleau-Ponty, Maurice. (2002 [1945]) *Phenomenology of Perception*. London: Routledge.
Meyer, Birgit. (2015) *Sensational Movies: Video, Vision, and Christianity in Ghana*. Berkeley, CA: University of California Press.
Mitchell, Jolyon and Plate, S. Brent. (eds.) (2007) *The Religion and Film Reader*. New York and London: Routledge.
Mitchell, W. J. T. (2005) *What Do Pictures Want? The Lives and Loves of Images*. Chicago: University of Chicago Press.
Morgan, David. (1999) *Visual Piety: A History and Theory of Popular Religious Images*. Berkeley, CA: University of California Press.
Morphy, Howard. (1991) *Ancestral Connections: Art and an Aboriginal System of Knowledge*. Chicago and London: University of Chicago Press.
Orsi, Robert. (2002 [1985]) *The Madonna of 115th Street: Faith and Community in Italian Harlem, 1880-1950*, 2nd ed. New Haven, CT: Yale University Press.
Pamuk, Orhan. (2001) *My Name is Red* (translated by Erdağ Göknar). New York: Alfred A. Knopf.
Plate, S. Brent. (2014) *A History of Religion in 5½ Objects: Bringing the Spiritual to Its Senses*. Boston: Beacon Press.
Promey, Sally. (ed.) (2014) *Sensational Religion: Sensory Cultures in Material Practice*. New Haven, CT: Yale University Press.
Sacks, Oliver. (1998 [1985]) *The Man Who Mistook His Wife for a Hat and Other Clinical Tales*. New York: Touchstone.
Singh, Anita. (2015) 'Aboriginal Art Unfit for Western Eyes,' *The Telegraph*, 2 May.
Stoller, Paul. (1989) *The Taste of Ethnographic Things: The Senses in Anthropology*. Philadelphia: University of Pennsylvania Press.
Turner, Edith. (2006) 'Advances in the Study of Spirit Experience: Drawing Together Many Threads,' *Anthropology of Consciousness*, 17 (2), 33–61.
Wilford, John Noble. (1983) 'Homer's Sea: Wine Dark?' *The New York Times*, 20 December.

Wilson, C. Roderick. (2012 [1994]) 'Seeing They See Not' in Young, D. E. and Goulet, J. (eds.), *Being Changed by Cross-Cultural Encounters: The Anthropology of Extraordinary Experience*. Ontario: University of Toronto Press, pp. 197–208.

Wolfson, E. R. (1994) *Through a Speculum that Shines: Vision and Imagination in Medieval Jewish Mysticism*. Princeton, NJ: Princeton University Press.

Dr Louise Child is a lecturer in myth, ritual and film studies at Cardiff University, UK, with research interests in altered states of consciousness including dreams, visions, mysticism, shamanism and possession trance, and their depictions in popular and indigenous films. She is a member of the British Association for the Study of Religion and has published on indigenous film in New Zealand for their journal. Her book *Tantric Buddhism and Altered States of Consciousness: Durkheim, Emotional Energy and Visions of the Consort* has recently been reissued in paperback by Routledge. She is currently working on a second book project, *Dreams, Vampires and Ghosts: Anthropological Perspectives on the Sacred and Psychology in Film and Television*.

Dr Aaron Rosen is Professor of Religion and Visual Culture and Director of the Henry Luce III Center for the Arts and Religion at Wesley Theological Seminary, Washington, DC. He was previously Senior Lecturer of Sacred Traditions and the Arts at King's College London, where he remains a visiting professor. Rosen began his career teaching at Yale, Oxford and Columbia Universities, after receiving his doctorate from the University of Cambridge. He is the author of *Art & Religion in the 21st Century*, *Imagining Jewish Art* and *Brushes with Faith*, and is at work on a monograph entitled *The Hospitality of Images*. His edited books include: *Religion and Art in the Heart of Modern Manhattan*; *Visualising a Sacred City: London, Art, and Religion*; and *Encounters: The Art of Interfaith Dialogue*. He regularly curates exhibitions and is the co-founder of the public arts project *Stations of the Cross*, which has been staged in London, New York, Washington, DC, and Amsterdam.

Section One
OBSCURITY

Chapter 1
Darkness Visible: The Art of Sam Winston

AARON ROSEN

In this interview, recorded in 2018, I speak with London-based artist Sam Winston about his artistic practice, which emphasises duration, experimentation and process. His previous works include Drawing Breath, *in which he drew a line for every single breath he took during an uninterrupted fifteen-hour period. Here, we speak about his recent works for the exhibition* Darkness Visible, *which invited audiences into a specially installed 'dark room' in the Southbank Centre, London in 2017-18. Drawing upon his experience creating works of art while blindfolded, and subsequently during days spent in complete darkness, the artist challenges viewers to 'see' darkness in new ways, disrupting traditional hierarchies of the senses, binaries of light and dark, and what it means to be a 'viewer.'*[1]

Aaron: Sam, you just returned from Norway, where I know you're thinking of doing a project. Given your interest in light, I imagine that was quite an interesting place with how radically light changes there during the year.

Sam: Well, one of the things I'm thinking about at the moment is liminal light, not just creating a body of work in liminal light, but also taking viewers to the smudge itself, to experience how different luminosities change the nature of the work (**Figure 1.1**).

Aaron: At the moment, though, you're very much immersed in doing dark works, right?

Sam: Right, I set up a dark space in the National Poetry Library [Southbank Centre, London]. I thought it would be really interesting to navigate spaces with your eyes shut, with a combination of vulnerability

---

1 A version of this interview appeared previously as: Rosen, Aaron. (2019) *Brushes with Faith: Reflections and Conversations on Contemporary Art.* Eugene, OR: Cascade.

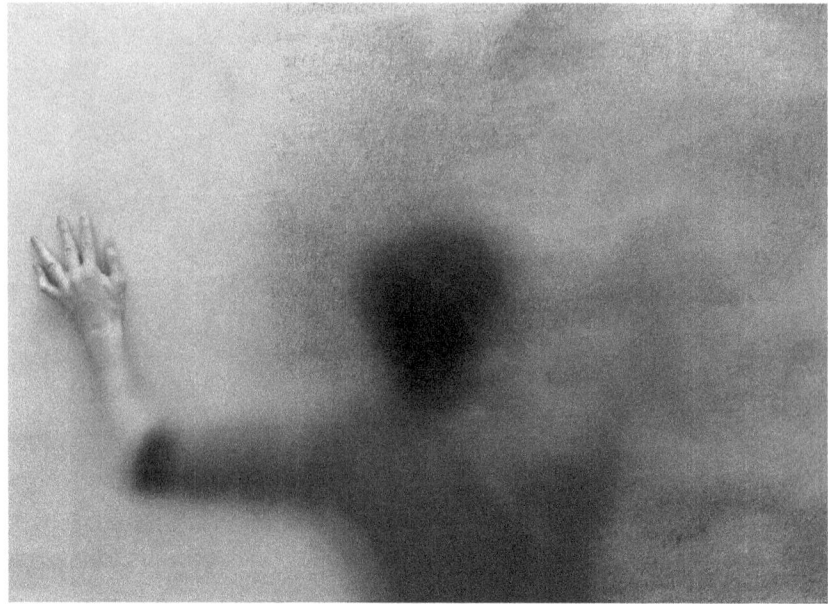

Figure 1.1 Sam Winston, *Erasure of Blind Drawing*, 2016. Photo: Andy Sewell / Sam Winston. Courtesy of and © Sam Winston.

and sensitivity. We've had a really strong response. I think we had over a thousand hours' worth of people standing in the dark. The hardest things to work with are the preconceived ideas about darkness being a place of evil, fear, torture or mental illness. But from the 170 or so remarks in the comments book, about eighty to ninety percent of them all referenced it being deeply restorative, deeply restful, un-scary, but also at times very transcendent. And three or four people said, 'I felt like a kid again.' A lot of people had quite an out-of-body experience. There wasn't an average. It was kind of marmite, it split people: either it was intense and they couldn't do it, or it was quite moving.

Aaron: Those reactions really seem to reveal the supremacy we give to vision among our senses. A lot of recent scholarship has explored how we've hierarchised our senses in various ways at different times and in different places. But certainly now, in the West, we place an immense empirical value on sight. When that's taken off the table, it's interesting to think about how we might validate our existence in different ways. When people say they have an out-of-body experience in your dark space it's interesting because of course the body's still there. So where is it that we think we exist when we aren't using sight to verify our experience?

Sam: I think the most threatening but also most appealing questions are who am I? and what am I? What happens when we can't lean on the predominant visual cue to have a 'sight body'? Using a 'touch body' or a 'sound body,' you begin to learn the new language of this space. For a while, people thought this was a project about blindness. For me it's about exploring this liminal transition between one sensory form and another, between sight and touch, or sight and sound. It's about trying to cope using different strategies in a completely different landscape, where you only have your ears to look. People going into the space might have five minutes of near panic, realising they're in a completely dark space, which is different than turning the lights out or having the curtain closed. Your eye is desperately looking for any frame of reference. And when it's not successful, the pay-off is a new freedom: you get out of the mode that you're existing in, and suddenly you have a new framework.

Aaron: It reminds me of pre-modern ideas about sight as a sort of extramission, that sight isn't so much received as sent out. In this case, it's like people in darkness send out their gaze but it can't latch onto anything. And you have to let that sense recognise its failure. But it's not blindness so much as the other senses being forced to 'do sight' in a different way. We aren't somehow instantly endowed with super-senses like superheroes. Our other senses try to create a totality of experience, and what constitutes a total experience gets re-conceptualised.

Sam: That's a perfect description. Another way of exploring it is visual acuity. I've been looking into the developmental stages that we have no conscious recollection of, the very early stages of sight. You are born at a stage in life where vision isn't up and running, so your first experience of the world is whilst vision itself is being built. And it seems like different stages of consciousness can be marked by how infants are able to discern between black and white and then between facial features and so on. It's a really beautiful primary language of shape and colour that is based around the visual acuity test. And that's what I'm exploring at the moment, whether viewers—consciously or unconsciously—can return to early vision, of say a week old. When you look at abstraction, is that part of what's going on? Can we trigger some of the first types of seeing that you ever did? So a part of this journey has led me into really thinking about the history of sight from a developmental perspective.

Aaron: That's so interesting. A mentor of mine, Doug Adams, used to talk about the process of learning to look at Abstract Expressionist paintings. For a lot of those painters, especially Rothko and Newman, who played a lot with latitude, the goal was to absorb you, to enclose you in the world of their painting. And if that entailed a lack of focus—akin to the sight of an infant—that actually meant getting it right. Maybe it's not incidental that Rothko was interested early in his career in childhood development. Another thing that interests me is how much we do for babies that's predicated on our own sensory experiences as adults. When we decorate a nursery, for example, we map our sensory experience onto babies, rather than trying to come closer to what it is that they are able to experience at a certain age.

Sam: I suppose you just resign yourself to the idea that basically you are passing on an inheritance that you received at a stage where you didn't have discretion either. When new people appear they have this massive download of information with very little filter. The issue of preconceptions ties back into the dark works. As I mentioned, I make a distinction between say blind drawing (**Figure 1.2**), which I've also done, and dark drawing,

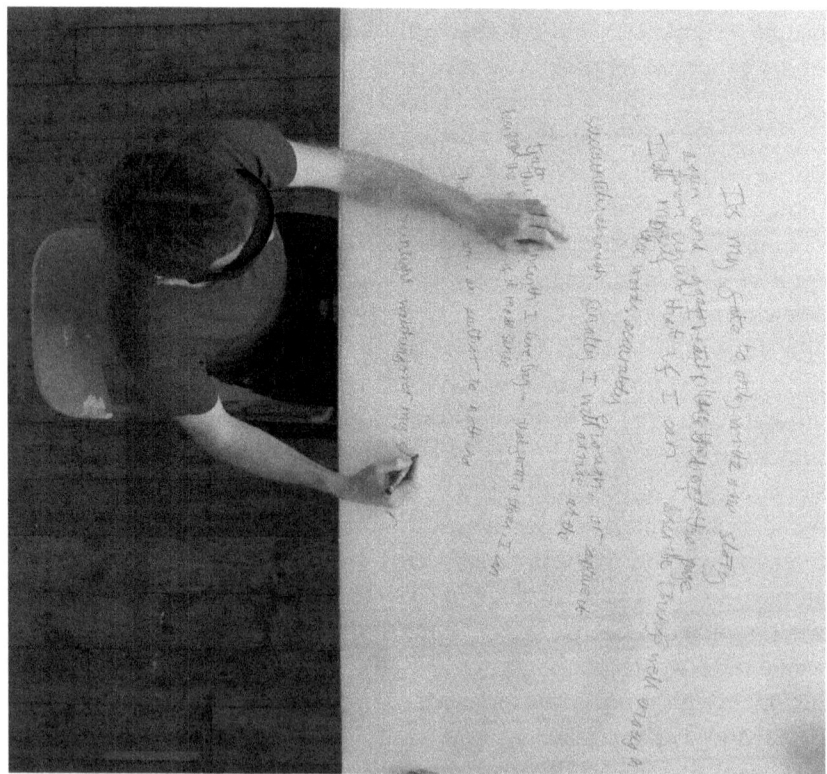

Figure 1.2 Sam Winston, *Blindfolded Text Drawing*, 2016. Photo: Andy Sewell / Sam Winston. Courtesy of and © Sam Winston.

which is a different experience. In blind drawing, you are visiting for a certain amount of time and whilst you're doing without sight, there's less of an altered state that happens. Whereas if you do a prolonged period in the dark, your consciousness and how you actually perceive and think is fundamentally different. Things like lucid dreaming become very prevalent. You're in a hypnagogic state; a dream space that you don't really get unless you start losing a sense of time after a couple days. I think there's an interesting connection in those experiences to early developmental stages of vision. I think it's not a coincidence that visitors said they were reminded of childhood. Not being a psychoanalyst, I can't quite say how that works, but it does seem that prolonged lucid dreaming brings up very early imagery, which is exactly why I'm interested in drawing from that space, which takes me back to a really early time (**Figure 1.3**).

Aaron: And maybe when people say they felt like children, that's simply because that's as far back as they can reach because of childhood amnesia, where we lose our early memories. So maybe when people are in the dark, what they're really tapping into are those experiences *behind* their memories.

Sam: But then there are also questions on the cultural level: how do you prepare people to go into a space that is fundamentally below

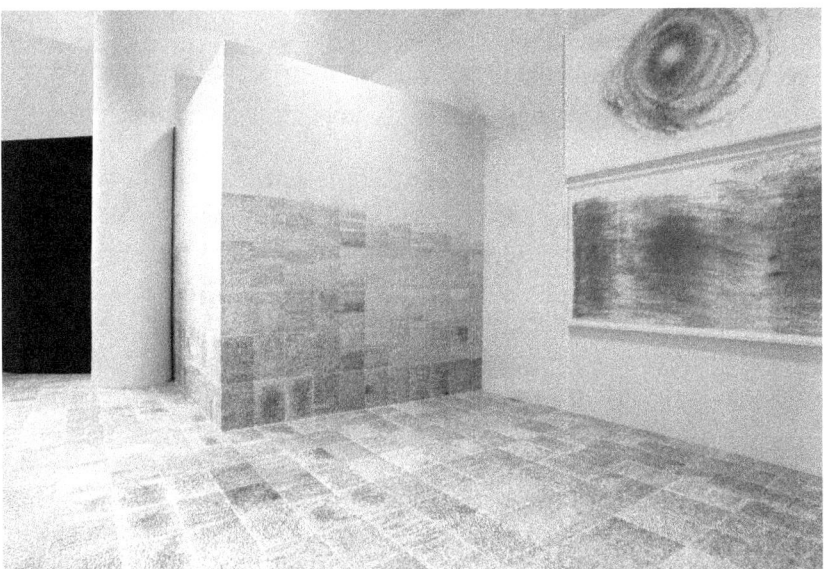

Figure 1.3 Sam Winston, *Darkness Visible*, 2017, installation view, Southbank Centre, London. Photo: Pietro Martini. Courtesy of and © Sam Winston.

consciousness? When we were doing the darkness exhibition at Whitechapel Gallery, most of our resources and time were spent building a useful narrative for audiences to explore the dark, and a comfort with the kinds of thoughts and emotions they might have. It's amazing how much energy was spent creating a story—that the dark is a very rich and fruitful place—which is completely true.

Aaron: What you're describing is a classic hermeneutic circle. I'm reminded of Heidegger and Gadamer insisting on acknowledging the value and force of the pre-understandings we bring to any act of interpretation. Your process acknowledges that people may not have a meaningful experience in the dark unless they're prepared to find it. I imagine one of the biggest challenges is to try and distil everything you've learned and try to give people an opportunity to have similar experiences, but without the luxury of spending a full week in utter darkness!

Sam: A lot of what I want to help visitors experience comes through my own process. At the moment I've been developing a series of drawings that involve looking at someone else, which in itself is quite hard. I think this also connects to early development. Children stare unabashedly for vast amounts of time because they're taking in this massive dataset. But culturally we eventually start to find this embarrassing. In the workshop we're developing, you draw the face blind, relying on your mind to pull up features in the right place. And then once the face is finished, you 'turn on' the eyes and create a replica of the blind drawing that you've done. In theory, this is all just looking, but each of those stages is a vastly different experience. It goes back to a really simple thing, which is looking at looking.

Aaron: In some ways, that workshop seems like a metaphor for your process more broadly. By analysing all of these different types of looking, you're trying to say something about the essence of looking. You're taking snapshots to get to a bigger picture.

Sam: Yeah, the work for me is always intuitive at first, then seeing where culture surfaces and how much of that experience you can translate, and what is acceptable to people. What I'm learning is that conversations with the health and safety and ticketing departments—convincing them that it's okay to let a thousand or two thousand people into a dark room without fire exit lighting—is also part of arts practice. There are norms in a public institution that say, 'this is what you need to do in a given situation.' But if you're trying to create a new experience, you have to take away some of the normative behaviours.

Aaron: Thinking about cultural and bureaucratic norms, I'm reminded of how much the social history of London is marked by evolving technologies of light. Gas streetlamps in the early nineteenth century completely changed public safety and discourses about criminality and poverty, while electrification in the late nineteenth and early twentieth centuries meant huge changes in commerce for places like Electric Avenue in Brixton. And now there's a big push for LED lights, which are meant to be more environmentally friendly since they use less energy. So there's this teleology of luminosity. Yet what you're doing is actually telling a story about *de*-illumination, about returning to the dark. How those stories intersect is fascinating. I'm also interested in how you see this project in relation to cultures with potentially different ideas about light and darkness.

Sam: In my research I'm definitely borrowing from various cultures. My friend who is a Tibetan monk does dark retreats and I know that there are a lot of indigenous practices like Native American sweat lodges, which focus on inwardness and darkness. Overall, there's a positive lexicon of light because we're all attracted to it, but the discourse of darkness tends to be about avoidance, aversion and distraction. People want to disturb the darkness with light. Part of what I'm doing is counterintuitive, because we live in an attention economy and a screen economy that's saturation rich.

Aaron: Emptiness and darkness often seem to be used pejoratively in our culture, constructed as qualities to eradicate. But illumination can also represent a type of loss. It's interesting that we're having this conversation on Earth Day, when we're being encouraged to turn off our lights. Not only does electric light use energy, of course, but light pollution obscures the stars and also alters animal migration. So, in a way, our desire for illumination can have damaging effects on our planet.

Sam: And of course it's not only affecting other species, we're reshaping our own behaviours. At a personal level, I've noticed how I use my eyes has changed over the last two decades. Especially with handheld devices, we're now constantly drifting between the screen and the natural landscape. For me, I still haven't got over the book, which induces its own kind of augmented reality! But now we're shifting into a world like that of Alice in Wonderland, in which you can go within the phone, within Instagram, within someone's feed, and then even go within that. There's this mysterious sense of depth and distance at the same time, which is becoming intuitive in its own way.

Aaron: So given all of these systemic challenges, how is it that you prepare people to step into a different type of space and experience, at odds with what they might be doing right before?

Sam: I realised I had to build up a series of strategies that I initially got from meditative practices. I realised you can't deal with the void by just saying, 'I'm going to pop into nothing.' You have to provide something for your body to do, an apparatus for certain types of thoughts. It's a very delicate balance where you're providing enough so you don't end up in a traumatic state, but not so much that you create just another routine. We have this amazing habit of turning our experience into what we were doing before.

Aaron: One of the things that strikes me as central to your practice is duration. On the one hand, you had to remain in the darkness for a certain amount of time to enable certain realisations, but you also had to know to go looking for that experience. So there's the durational arc of your creative practice as well.

Sam: I tend to put the whole narrative of a project's creation—with the time and the effort and the sacrifice involved—into the final thing. I've spent a couple of decades being a visual artist and to spend a week without being able to reference what I'm doing and to look at it meant that it was probably the hardest project I've ever done. Relinquishing sight meant a loss of the visual story. When you're doing the work in complete darkness, there's a real pronounced longing to see something, and you build up quite an elaborate narrative about what the thing looks like. You know that there's a thing there and it exists and it has a whole, and the question is how to get the audience to experience that.

Aaron: The sense of longing that you're talking about is so powerful. Do you think consciously of that having a theological dimension? I know you're quite literate in a number of different religious and cultural contexts. Do you find theological analogies useful, or do you find yourself fighting that kind of language?

Sam: Well, I continue learning. I'm literate in that language, as you say, and I've been able to access religious experience in different traditions. Over time I developed this sense of what I'm aiming towards in different contexts. I was doing a talk for the MA at Wimbledon College of Arts recently and someone asked me, 'Are you a monk?' I've never framed my work in that way because it explains it in far too simplistic a term. I don't fight it, but I try not to give frameworks that people are already going to assume about the work, which is hard because generally people won't do something until they've been told what the thing is. Even just saying something is an art exhibition means people pull up fifty art exhibitions they've been to before. If I find myself in a particularly religious setting, then I feel very much drawn to questioning the institutional side of art.

But within the art context, I find myself pushing against the norms of the art world, looking for a way to experience the transcendent, or something without form.

Aaron: So it sounds like ironically there's more latitude for you to open the door to theology when you're in a museum or gallery context because there's no risk that it will be the totalising frame by which people see their experience.

Sam: Yeah, in some ways, that's because of the age of this form. Art—in the way we understand it presently—is a baby in comparison to spiritual life. I do think at one point it will be studied and considered in a similar way one would do theology now. But I'm well aware that I'm walking very much around your territory here.

Aaron: It's okay, I'll give you a day pass into the divinity faculty....

Dr Aaron Rosen is Professor of Religion and Visual Culture and Director of the Henry Luce III Center for the Arts and Religion at Wesley Theological Seminary, Washington, DC. He was previously Senior Lecturer of Sacred Traditions and the Arts at King's College London, where he remains a visiting professor. Rosen began his career teaching at Yale, Oxford and Columbia Universities, after receiving his doctorate from the University of Cambridge. He is the author of *Art & Religion in the 21st Century*, *Imagining Jewish Art* and *Brushes with Faith*, and is at work on a monograph entitled *The Hospitality of Images*. His edited books include: *Religion and Art in the Heart of Modern Manhattan*; *Visualising a Sacred City: London, Art, and Religion*; and *Encounters: The Art of Interfaith Dialogue*. He regularly curates exhibitions and is the co-founder of the public arts project *Stations of the Cross*, which has been staged in London, New York, Washington, DC, and Amsterdam.

Chapter 2

Visibly Invisible: Muslim Women in Twenty-first Century Political Cartoons

TAHNIA AHMED

Britain has a long history of political cartooning, remarkable for its incisive commentary and largely unfettered freedom of expression. Francis Carruthers Gould (1844–1925) became the first British cartoonist for a newspaper in 1888, the *Pall Mall Gazette*, followed by major figures such as David Low (1891–1963) for *The Evening Standard*, and John Tenniel (1820–1914) for *Punch*, the legendary humour magazine (Seymour-Ure 2001: 333). This rich satirical culture continues today, with political cartoonists such as Steve Bell, Gerald Scarfe and Peter Brookes household names in the country. As Lewis Perry Curtis, Jr. states, the importance of the political cartoon lies in the:

> reciprocal relationship between those who create it and those who consume it.... As much as any of their contemporaries...[cartoonists]...live and practice within ideology, drawing literally and figuratively on prejudices that already lurk or inhere in their audiences. (1997: x)

This has been particularly true of Britain, in which most major newspapers have easily discernible political commitments and target audiences. The publications I examine in this essay, for example, broadly speaking run the gamut from left-wing to right-wing: *The Independent* (and *iNews*), *The Times*, *The Daily Telegraph*, *The Daily Mail* and *The Sun*. Based on the way in which political cartoons both seek and presuppose their readers' agreement, they are a profoundly illuminating source for gauging responses to pressing social issues.

This chapter examines the portrayal of Muslim women in British political cartoons since the fall of the Afghanistan government, the Taliban, in 2001 as a consequence of the United States led 'War on Terror,' supported by the United Kingdom. This was hardly the first time that British cartoonists turned their eye toward Muslims. The publication of Salman Rushdie's novel *The Satanic Verses* in 1988, which retold episodes from the life of the Prophet Muhammad, sparked outrage in the Muslim community across the world, stoked by a *fatwa* issued by Ayatollah Khomeini, calling for the killing of Rushdie (Murtagh 1989). In the UK, the *fatwa* provoked intense debate surrounding freedom of expression and Muslim identity, with many framing it as struggle between Islamic and Western values. Cartoonists took note, often creating caricatures of angry Muslim men, images which would be renewed and reconfigured in the wake of the terror attacks of 11 September 2001 and especially the London bombings of 7 July 2005. Women are notably absent in most cartoons stemming from the controversy over *The Satanic Verses*. The unseating of the Taliban, frequently presented and rationalised as a liberation of Afghan women, catalysed a new wave of images of female Muslims, not only abroad but at home.

The image of the veil—in various forms—lies at the centre of these images, and the perception of Muslim women more generally. Religious covering in Islam remains greatly misunderstood, and it is worth offering some context before proceeding with our examination of images. Many Muslims believe that it is a religious obligation for female Muslims to veil themselves, based on several verses in the Qur'an, such as Q33:59:

> Prophet, tell your wives, your daughters, and women believers to make their outer garments hang low over them a so as to be recognized and not insulted: God is most forgiving, most merciful.

There are a multitude of interpretations of just what the Qur'an means in relation to the practice of veiling. The most common form of veiling across the globe is the headscarf, commonly known as *hijab* or *khimar*, with which a Muslim woman covers her hair. In addition to the headscarf, many women also choose to wear a cloak over their clothes known as a *jilbab* or *abaya*, often worn by women in the Middle East. The *chador*, mainly worn by women in Iran, is a cloak covering the entire body, which is held closed at the front. Other Muslim women wear the *burqa*, a one-piece veil covering the entire face and body—mostly associated with women in Afghanistan— or the *niqab*, a veil covering the face, leaving the eyes clear. One interesting example of a Muslim woman's decision to wear the headscarf is found in

Myfanwy Franks' research regarding Caucasian Muslim converts. One of the women interviewed, Miriam, speaks about her husband's ambivalence at her decision to wear the headscarf. Miriam cites the Bosnian War as the main reason for her decision to do so. In this example, Miriam goes against the prevailing view of the dominant Muslim male forcing her to veil. Furthermore, Miriam chooses to wear the headscarf in part because her physical appearance is not so different to those who were persecuted in Bosnia on the grounds of their faith (Franks 2000: 925).

THE POWER OF THE GAZE

Michel Foucault famously argued that the gaze constitutes a form of power. In surveillance, the power of authority is 'visible and unverifiable' (Foucault 2008: 6). Meyda Yegenoglu helpfully builds upon this Foucauldian paradigm to articulate the latent power dynamics at stake in debates over the (in)visibility of Muslim women's bodies. She calls attention to the ways in which the body of the Muslim woman, or *Muslimah*, is fixated upon by the colonialist Westerner. Rendered opaque to the colonial gaze, the veiled Muslimah 'is both an object of hostility and an object of fascination and these are expressed as a continual quest for knowledge' (Yegenoglu 1998: 110). In this way, the feminine body that is not veiled is presented as the norm, whilst the veiled female body represents an oppressed and subjugated woman who embodies all that is wrong with Islam.

> [T]he representation of woman as tradition and as the essence of the Orient, made it all the more important to lift the veil, *for unveiling and thereby modernizing the woman of the Orient signified the transformation of the Orient itself.* (Yegenoglu 1998: 99; emphasis original)

I argue that cartoon images of veiled Muslim women convey messages of political and cultural deception, suspicion and oppression against women. Exotic and alluring, yet at the same time dangerous and subversive, media representations of Muslim women are multifaceted and complex. In the political cartoons examined below, I find that the *burqa/niqab* iconographies are used interchangeably to make a wider point about the *veiling of the face*, as opposed to veiling of the hair, which is seemingly deemed acceptable. The *burqa/niqab* is perceived as a self-conscious marker of subversion of Western ideals such as democracy, free speech and the freedom of movement for women. Moreover, there is an assumption that the *burqa/niqab* only serve to repress one's femininity, disregarding the different reasons and meanings behind a woman wearing it, thereby creating an illusion of the Muslimah who is oppressed and voiceless, in need of saving from the Muslim male (Fernandez 2009: 272). Such portrayals of the Muslimah are instructive because they are also a comment on the Muslim male and the perception that he is 'the barbaric controlling Other' (Fernandez 2009: 275). I look at how this is translated in visual culture and the implications of these tropes in the wider context relating to perceptions of gender, national identity and violence.

The Muslimah is figured as blind, someone to whom social norms do not apply. If she cannot see, she cannot object to being stared at. Gili Hammer's study of blind women offers an interesting point of comparison. 'While the gaze sexualizes,' Hammer suggests, 'staring dehumanizes.' Blindness—or in our case purported blindness—accentuates the visibility of the subject (Hammer 2016: 418). On the one hand, the *burqa/niqab* serves to deflect the gaze, averting sexualisation and seemingly promising invisibility. And yet, in a context in which her garments set her apart from most other members of the British public, the Muslimah becomes the object of stares, someone whom the non-Muslim viewer implicitly identifies as a forcibly covered subject in need of unveiling and 'liberation.' The veiled Muslimah, and by extension all Muslim women, become *visibly invisible*.

MUSLIMS IN BRITAIN

Calls to be able to wear the *burqa/niqab* have proved to be major points of contention in Britain, sparking debate surrounding where—and whether—the Muslim community fits into British society (Deedes 2006). Muslims in Britain are not a monolithic group. They represent a constellation of different ethnic, cultural and linguistic groups. This makes it highly problematic to speak about 'the Muslim community' in Britain, as often happens. Demonstrating this, in their analysis of the 2011 Census, The Muslim Council of Britain (MCB) observed that the ethnic diversity of the Muslim population in Britain is on the increase as those who describe themselves as 'Black African,' 'Black other' and 'Asian other' have risen in population numbers. Notwithstanding this fact, a large part of today's Muslim presence can be traced back to Commonwealth immigration from South Asia in the 1950s, of which Pakistanis make up the largest single ethnic group at just over one million in the 2011 Census (MCB 2015: 24). Many of these South Asian immigrants came to satisfy the demand for industrial workers in Britain, with their wives and children joining them from around the 1970s onwards (Modood 2006: 37).

Tariq Modood recounts his own experience of growing up in Britain where he was brought up to 'never deny that we are Pakistanis (later this became Asian, and then Muslim)' (Modood 2005: 4), showing the fluid and multidimensional character of Muslim identity in Britain. Precisely because of this, Modood's focus on discourses surrounding race and ethnicity provides a more useful insight than an historical analysis which depends upon a single, static definition of Muslim identity. He notes that whilst the Jewish and the Sikh communities are legally recognised as ethnic groups, the Muslim community does not enjoy such status. This is due to the fact that, much like Christianity, Islam is from its beginning defined as universal and not ethnocentric. Hence, before religious discrimination was recognised in legislation in 2003 (*Employment Equality Regulations*), the focus on race and ethnicity meant that though Muslims may have been discriminated against as Muslims, they often had to reference being Pakistani or Arab, for example, to seek protection (Modood 2005: 38). Therefore, the experience of a Muslim immigrant is more likely to be predominantly bound up with his/her race, rather than religion. Modood criticises the approach taken from the 1970s through the early 1980s of 'political blackness,' in which Britons fell into two categories: black or white. This meant those who fell in the 'black' category included any people 'who were potential victims of colour racism.' Such an approach was at first embraced and then later rejected by 'Asian political activists' who sought 'a more particular ethnic or religious identity rather than this all-inclusive non-whiteness' (Modood 2006: 41).

Today, there are over 2.7 million Muslims living in England and Wales, making up 4.8% of the population. Of this, just under 1.3m are women (MCB 2015: 40). Interestingly, the MCB found that 73% of Muslims in Britain 'consider British to be their only national identity' (MCB 2015: 34) even though over half of them were born outside of the UK. While there are, to be sure, overarching issues facing Muslim men and women alike, they often face and respond to questions of cultural difference in different ways. According to Tahir Abbas:

> Young Muslim women have been shown to better engage with the theological, political and social pressures placed on their identities as British-born and Muslim people. Without doubt, it is reasonably well confirmed that Muslim women outperform their male counterparts in higher education, and are more successful in negotiating issues of ethnicity, identity and high profile religious minority status (Abbas 2008: 292).

If anything, this makes the treatment of Muslim women by British cartoonists even more problematic. Rather than looking to how these women articulate their own identity, cartoonists frequently resort to the stereotype of a Muslim woman who is unwilling—or unable—to embrace ideas such as gender equality, democracy and transparency, which are considered fundamental British values. I now turn my attention to specific examples from recent cartoons, which foreground these tensions between perception and reality.

VEILED, UNNAMED AND OPPRESSED

Following the Bank of England's decision to replace the image of Elizabeth Fry on the £5 banknote with that of Winston Churchill (Peachey 2013) there was a public outcry that there would no longer be any females featured other than the Queen (Criado-Perez 2013). In a separate interview a few months later, the Business Secretary, Vince Cable, likened the Bank of England to the Taliban in relation to its fiscal policies (Saul 2013). Commenting on the subsequent decision to feature Jane Austen on £10 banknotes ('Jane Austen' 2013) and the Taliban comparison, **Peter Brookes' 'New Jane Austen £10 Note (as designed by Vince Cable)'** (*The Times*, 25 July 2013)[1] shows Jane Austen (the ringlets of hair and eyes in the likeness of the portrait by James Andrews from 1869) wearing the *niqab*. The use of the *niqab* in the cartoon is contentious because it explicitly connects the Muslim religion with gender inequality. Austen appears in the foreground dressed in a black *niqab*, writing the well-known opening words of *Pride and Prejudice*—'It is a truth universally acknowledged, that a single man in possession of a good fortune, must be in want of a wife'—which have been amended to refer to the 'Taleban' (sic). This is all despite the fact that the Taliban or Islam have never had any influence in the Bank of England's decision on who should appear on English banknotes. Thus, Brookes' 'New Jane Austen £10 Note [...]' illustrates the perception of the Muslimah in a *niqab* equating to something that is un-British and alien. Through using the stereotype of the veiled Muslimah, there is a presumption that the *niqab* represses both femininity and the ability to participate fully in British society. Brookes attempts to highlight anti-feminist aspects of British society through portraying Austen *as a Muslim*, insinuating that to be so is to be anti-feminist. Thus, in order to combat the prejudice that

---

[1] The new £10 note came into circulation in July 2017.

women face in British society, one must accentuate anti-Islamic prejudice. By reversing the message of the cartoon, the reader understands that were the woman unveiled she would undoubtedly be un-oppressed and fully exercise her rights as a British citizen. In this way, the image almost goes against its artistic intent: by depicting Austen in such a manner on the banknote, she is rendered invisible and almost nonexistent. To view Austen wearing the *niqab* is to not see her at all.

The idea of the Muslim male as 'the barbaric controlling Other' as mentioned above is exemplified in **Dave Brown's uncaptioned image** (*The Independent*, 3 August 2005). In this image, the then counter-terrorism minister, Hazel Blears, is caricatured in such a manner as to make her seem unattractive. Against the silhouette of a mosque, two Muslim men look on at Blears in distaste, one of whom comments: 'Y'know...Just occasionally... Enforcing the burka doesn't seem like a bad idea!' Here, Brown refers to the broad powers granted to the police to stop and search anyone without cause.[2] This led to feelings of resentment amongst Muslim communities who felt that they were being racially profiled by the police, especially following the 7/7 attacks ('Blears seeks' 2005). Here, the *burqa* acts both as a way to shield the men—as well as wider society—from the sight of Blears' ostensibly unattractive physical appearance, as well as serving to disempower her from implementing her unpopular counter-terrorism measures. The image insinuates that there is power for those who can be seen, whilst those who are cloaked are left powerless. Furthermore, that the women in Brookes' and Brown's images are both not even Muslim demonstrates the idea of Islam as a tool to stealthily take over Britain in such a manner as to make *all* women invisible.

This idea can also be seen in **Peter Brookes' 'Meanwhile, in downtown Kabul...'** (*The Times*, 16 November 2001), published following the US-led invasion of Afghanistan in 2001, which resulted in the collapse of the Taliban regime after five years of brutal rule. This led to significant changes allowing Afghan women the right to vote, work and be educated (*Constitution of Afghanistan* 2004). Perhaps most famously, women no longer had to wear the *burqa* as had been enforced by the Taliban regime (RAWA n.d.). 'Meanwhile, in downtown Kabul...' depicts two women in heels and fishnets, wearing short dresses. An Afghan male street seller in traditional clothing (known as a *perahon tunban*) who whistles at them receives an angry retort from one of the women to 'BURKA OFF, MATE!'

---

2 These powers were repealed under the *Protection of Freedoms Act 2012* and replaced with Article 3 of *The Terrorism Act 2000 (Remedial) Order 2011*.

The juxtaposition of the women in Western clothing against the street seller in traditional clothing suggests how their attire reflects their contrasting attitudes towards gender. By celebrating the liberation of women in such a way, the cartoon suggests that if the status quo was to remain, the women would not have been noticed by the street seller for their beauty and neither would the women have the ability to speak up for themselves against inappropriate behaviour.

The cartoon illustrates how women's rights were seen as such a central issue, viewing the war in Afghanistan as a means to liberate Afghan women. At the same time, 'New Jane Austen £10 Note [...]' and 'Meanwhile, in downtown Kabul...' both demonstrate a conflation of the Taliban with the wider issue of women's rights as symbolised by the *burqa/niqab*. For example, 'New Jane Austen £10 Note [...]' appropriates the imagery of a woman in a black *niqab*, comparing Britain to the collapsed Taliban state in Afghanistan where women are not allowed to participate fully in society, insinuating the demise of an egalitarian Western society. The cartoon's focus on the veiled woman serves to emphasise her alien status in a democratic country. In fact, this line of thinking shares common ground with the Taliban's view of women: those who did *not* veil had no place in such a political system, demonstrating how a woman's right to participate in society is so often predicated on whether or not she wears the veil. Moreover, the terms employed such as 'Taliban' and 'jihadist' in relation to the Bank of England are interesting in understanding the message conveyed by Cable and the official policy quoted in *The Independent* article (Saul 2013). In using such terminology, there is a clear intention to portray the Bank of England as the enemy, starkly presented as the aggressor because of its policies towards banks. 'New Jane Austen £10 Note [...]' having been printed twelve years after the collapse of the Taliban regime, demonstrates the impact of 9/11 and the War on Terror on more recent perceptions of the Muslim community both in Britain and abroad.

THE FACE VEIL: TO BAN OR NOT TO BAN?

Depicting a woman in *niqab* being chased by a policeman on a topless beach in St Tropez, **Matt's uncaptioned image** (*Daily Telegraph*, 12 April 2011) shows the irony of the newly imposed French ban on face veils in public whilst people are free to (not) wear anything they like—providing it is not the *burqa* or *niqab*. The cartoon shows a topless mother shielding her child's eyes from the veiled woman, further adding to the absurdity of the situation. The idea that a woman covered head to toe would be deemed too explicit for the child to witness serves to break down negative perceptions and stereotypes. This is contrary to the message of the previous cartoons examined, wherein the actual *burqa/niqab* garment makes the Muslimah visible. By choosing to veil herself in such a manner at the beach, she has intentionally broken the law, whilst also offending the sensibilities of the French general public. The cartoon attempts to highlight how the ban created further inequalities and restrictions, rather than dissolve them as purported,[3] echoing the sentiments of *The Times* editorial on the issue of the face veil ban, that 'it is surely an irony to seek to defend liberal European values of tolerance and sexual freedom by restricting the freedom of women to dress as they wish' ('In Your Face' 2011).

The decision by Belgium and France to ban face veils in public sparked debate about a potential ban in Britain. Resisting calls for a ban to be imposed, the then Immigration Minister, Damian Green, stated that it would be '"un-British" and run contrary to the conventions of a tolerant and mutually respectful society' (Hennessy 2010). **Peter Schrank's uncaptioned cartoon** (*The Independent*, 19 July 2010) depicts an elderly Caucasian man sitting on a park bench, looking on at the passers-by dressed in summer clothing. A thought bubble above his head reads 'Sometimes I rather wish it could be made compulsory' in response to the newspaper's headline in his hands, 'No burka ban for Britain.' The image illustrates the issue from a different perspective; the enforcement of the *burqa/niqab* on *non*-Muslims would be welcome so that those who, according to the elderly man, dress inappropriately are made to wear more modest attire. At the same time, perhaps Schrank is also conveying how such ideas are outdated and regressive as symbolised by the juxtaposition of an elderly man regarding a much younger generation. Therefore, Schrank exposes the irony of orthodox Muslim views on veiling being in line with retrograde gender attitudes held by members of the elderly Caucasian population. This is in contrast to that of the more 'tolerant' younger Caucasian generation; if the man sitting on the bench was in fact young he would be more accepting of the diversity of attire. Similar to Matt's cartoon, Schrank depicts an absurd situation in which (non-Muslim) Britons are shown to dress in a way that seems distasteful and yet are seemingly more accepted by society than a woman dressed in a *burqa* or *niqab*.

---

3 In his state of the nation speech, French President Sarkozy argued that the face veil meant women were 'prisoners behind a screen, cut off from all social life, deprived of all identity. That's not our idea of freedom.' See Chrisafis (2009).

Muslim Women in Political Cartoons   35

In July 2010, the then Environment Secretary, Caroline Spelman, shared her views on the *burqa* in an interview, stating that 'for a woman it is empowering to be able to choose each morning when you wake up what you wear' (Slack 2010). Her support for the *burqa* and the use of the word 'empowering' in relation to it made national headlines.[4] **Mac's 'Doris, love. How would you like to feel empowered?'** (*Daily Mail*, 20 July 2010), depicts a Caucasian couple at breakfast, where the husband poses the question to his wife (**Figure 2.1**).

In her survey of the perception of veiled women, Sonya Fernandez argues that the dichotomous presentation of the West vs Islam leads to a:

> focus on gender issues such as veiling, honour killing and forced marriage [...which act...] as the perfect prop for justifying the forceful imposition of western values on the cultural Other, by pointing to the oppression of women in Other cultures while simultaneously ignoring the oppression of women within the dominant culture (Fernandez 2009: 271).

The scene presented to the reader lends credence to this argument: the husband sits at the kitchen table, reading a newspaper headlined 'BURKAS

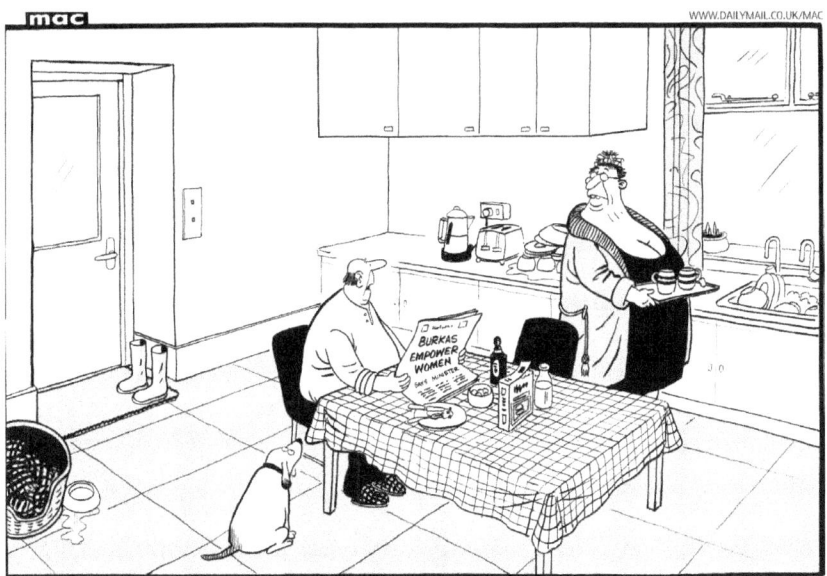

'Doris, love. How would you like to feel empowered?'

Figure 2.1 Mac, 'Doris, love. How would you like to feel empowered?' *Daily Mail*, 20 July 2010.

4 See Prince (2010) and Alibhai-Brown (2010).

EMPOWER WOMEN SAYS MINISTER', whilst his wife Doris carries a tray with two mugs over to a sink full of dirty crockery. Their situation is ironic: Doris, a non-Muslim, fulfils the stereotype of a disempowered wife, literally stuck in the kitchen. By posing the question to Doris, perhaps the husband wishes to trick her into further disempowerment by making her wear the *burqa* and ensuring her subservience to him. Further still, despite it not being incumbent in Islam to veil in the presence of one's husband (as well as certain other male family members), the fact that Doris's husband wishes his wife to do so indicates that perhaps he does not find her physically attractive and wishes to remedy this by getting her to wear the *burqa*, thus echoing the sentiments in Dave Brown's uncaptioned image (*The Independent*, 3 August 2005). By regarding the *burqa* as a way of empowering women (as the cartoon suggests she does) Spelman disregards the underlying issues of gender inequality the *burqa* represents. Mac's 'Doris, love. How would you like to feel empowered?' raises further questions about the different ways gender inequality exists and the focus on particular cultures in relation to this issue. On the whole, the cartoons perpetuate the idea that such inequalities are almost exclusive to Muslims in Britain, ignoring the fact that gender inequalities exist amongst non-Muslims too.

Matt's **'And don't be late tomorrow, it's the school photo…'** (*Daily Telegraph*, 17 September 2013) responds to Birmingham Metropolitan College lifting its eight-year ban on *burqas* following a petition instigated by a complaint from a prospective student (NUS Black Students' Campaign 2014). The cartoon shows a male teacher instructing his students—all of whom wear the *niqab*—to ensure they arrive in time for the school photo tomorrow. Published two years after the ban in France, 'And don't be late tomorrow […]' seems to view the issue of veiling from a different angle. The reader is presented with an image of an all-female, all-Muslim class who are taught by a Caucasian male. The juxtaposition of a *niqab*-wearing Muslimah being willingly educated in a Western educational establishment deftly illustrates the British approach of 'tolerance' towards such issues, where apparent contradictions and conflicts between different cultures are absorbed. This is reflected in the ambivalence in this cartoon that is not found in Matt's uncaptioned image (*Daily Telegraph*, 12 April 2011). For example, 'And don't be late tomorrow […]' demonstrates the apparent ease of the interaction between the teacher and the veiled students. Importantly, the act of veiling does not pose any barriers to the students' education, nor to the teacher being able to perform his job properly. Therefore, the fact that their faces cannot be fully seen does not mean that the girls do not wish to partake fully in society, nor do they believe the veil stops them from doing so.

Whilst Brown and Brookes focus on the way the face veil can be a tool for disempowerment and to cloak one's looks, Matt demonstrates that this is not necessarily true. By educating themselves, the schoolgirls are becoming empowered, where the issue of physical beauty is not something that they are concerned with. At the same time, the cartoon seems to echo fears that lifting the ban on face veils gives way to an interpretation of Islam that does not accept diversity and encourages gender inequality. This is symbolised in the image of very young Muslim girls (the text 'CLASS 8C' on the noticeboard in the background indicates that these girls are 12–13 years of age) who seemingly accept this inequality by choosing to wear the *niqab*. Thus, 'And don't be late tomorrow [...]' challenges the reader to make up her own mind as to what allowing the face veil in the classroom means in relation to British society: is it a question of religious freedom or is this a sign that Islam and British identity are incompatible?

THE *BURQA* AS DISGUISE

Aside from the gender equality issue, another trend emerges: presenting the *burqa* and *niqab* as tools for deception. **Peter Brookes' 'Silly Burka...'** (*The Times*, 5 November 2013) is a trio of images of the same woman wearing a blue *burqa*. The cloaked woman has a red ministerial box, indicating her prominent position in government. In the final image, the red box is lifted to reveal the minister's leopard-skin heels. The minister depicted is Theresa May, the then Home Office minister, well-known for her leopard-skin shoes and whose remit included anti-terror legislation. May was criticised when terror suspect, Mohammed Ahmed Mohamed, managed to escape wearing a *burqa* despite strict restrictions (known as TPIMs or terrorism prevention and investigation measures) placed on him (Dodd 2013). The caption suggests May's frustration and embarrassment at the situation, while the image suggests a shirking of ministerial responsibility but also a sense of naivety: May attempts to replicate the apparent ease with which Mohamed was able to escape the authorities by wearing a *burqa* to avoid having to confront the issue in her capacity as Home Office minister. However, her striking heels and red box give her away.

Commenting on the same topic, **Matt's 'Wait till I catch that cat...'** (8 November 2013, *Daily Telegraph*), shows a cat (distinguishable by its tail) in plain view, wearing a *niqab*. However, the cat's owner seems not to see it as he complains about the damage done to his armchair by his pet. Both images reflect incredulity at the way Mohamed was able to evade the authorities. Brookes' image takes a more nuanced political view, whilst Matt focuses on the simplicity of Mohamed's escape. In similar vein, following the fall of Tripoli into rebel hands, **Matt's uncaptioned image** (*Daily Telegraph*, 30 August 2011) shows a woman wearing a *niqab*, wearing sunglasses and decorated in military medals and epaulettes. The woman walks past a sign: 'SEARCH FOR GADDAFI', the implication being that 'she' is actually Colonel Muammar Gaddafi, the former Libyan dictator, evading capture by donning the *niqab*. Illustrating a sense of mistrust and suspicion towards the face veil, these cartoons present it as a form of disguise, where the cat, May and Gaddafi seek to evade culpability for their actions by (ab)using the Islamic veil.

Such sentiments are echoed in **Brighty's 'Nothing to hide'** (*The Sun*, 16 September 2013), published in response to a court trial during which a Muslimah argued against having to take the face veil off when giving evidence (Morrison 2013). The cartoon visualises the defendant in a *niqab* in the witness box; the angle from which the reader sees the Muslimah makes her tower over the reader in an almost intimidating manner. This, along with the simple statement coming from the Muslimah that she has 'Nothing to hide,' convey to the reader the very opposite: this particular woman does in fact have something to hide, and it is not just her face.

The portrayal of the veiled Muslimah is often as an unnamed, unidentifiable individual. Within this, a process of disembodiment and dehumanisation occurs when it comes to the 'typical' Muslimah, which serves to emphasise the *burqa/niqab* as a tool for oppression, but also disassociates the reader from the object, turning the Muslimah into an Other. This is in stark contrast to May and Gaddafi, two political figures, who are given the 'privilege' of being instantly recognisable in the cartoons, despite their attempts at going undercover. This seems to contradict the idea that the *burqa/niqab* is a tool for suppressing one's individuality; rather, it suggests that the *burqa/niqab* is unsuccessful in doing so because there are other ways of expressing one's self—be it high heels or epaulettes. On the other hand, perhaps this signifies how the *burqa/niqab* should be seen as one of the myriad ways in which women choose to *clothe* themselves (as opposed to veiling themselves in a way that is disconnected to any other garments that they choose to wear with or without it).

Brian Klug theorises that 'new antisemitism' works upon 'an *a priori* prejudice that revolves around a fiction, a figment of what Jews are like' (Klug 2012: 135) In other words, it is a predisposed perception of Jews that *then* seeks substantiation with the wider world. Drawing from this, Modood and Nasar Meer argue that the same occurs with the Muslim community today (Meer and Modood 2009: 339). If views presented in political cartoons are symptomatic of a wider presumed consensus, as I assert they are, it follows that this informs the reader of pre-existing stereotypes and views which are then built upon in these images. From the cartoons looked at here, there is an assumption that the very act of veiling is born out of a desire to prevent the Muslimah from being able to participate fully in British society by causing her to be unseen or unheard in a way somewhat similar to how women were treated under Taliban rule in Afghanistan.

WHOSE VALUES?

The Charlie Hebdo shooting that took place in Paris on 7 January 2015, in which twelve people died, was carried out by the Yemeni branch of Al Qaeda (Al Qaeda in the Arabian Peninsula—AQAP). AQAP claimed that the motive behind the attack was the publication of satirical cartoons of the Prophet by the *Charlie Hebdo* newspaper ('Al-Qaeda in Yemen' 2015). In response to the attack, the hashtag 'Je suis Charlie' was used in social media to demonstrate solidarity with the victims. **Peter Brookes' 'New UK Poll…'** (*The Times*, 26 February 2015) depicts a Muslimah wearing a *niqab*, walking along a street carrying a handbag in one hand and a Tesco carrier bag in the other. Crucially, she wears a white vest over her *abaya* which reads 'JE SUIS 75% CHARLIE.' The statement refers to the results of a survey for BBC Radio 4 Today of 1,000 Muslims in Britain in which 27% agreed with the statement: 'I have some sympathy for the motives behind the attacks on Charlie Hebdo in Paris' (ComRes 2015: 14). Brookes picks up on the significant number of Muslims who sympathised with the attack, demonstrating how the Muslimah wearing the face veil is often used to symbolise the entire British Muslim community. This image also demonstrates how there is an expectation of British Muslims by the wider British public to speak out against attacks that are carried out by other Muslims around the world. Despite the fact that the overwhelming majority of those polled (62%) said they disagreed with the statement (ComRes 2015: 18), Brookes' cartoon draws attention to the minority who did agree. The act of veiling serves to unmask what the person *really* thinks; by wearing the *niqab* along with the vest it undermines the poll results. The insinuation being that one who dresses in such a manner cannot possibly be part of the 75%, thereby rendering the poll results invalid. In many ways, the image conveys a sense of incredulity that there exists diversity of thought and opinion within the British Muslim community, especially in relation to this particular topic. This suggests that were the same poll to be conducted with non-Muslims, there would undoubtedly be unanimous disagreement with such a statement.

Our final image is **Ben Jennings' 'This is what I'm talking about people! The "Burka" is an affront to our Christian values!'** (*i News*, 29 April 2017). The cartoon comments on the UK Independence Party (UKIP) proposals to ban the face veil as part of their 2015 general election campaign (Elgot 2017). In the first scene, the party leader, Paul Nuttall, points to the backs of two women cloaked in black as they walk along the street, exclaiming the words in the caption. The second box then shows the two women turn around, one of whom asks Nuttall, 'What's that, luv?' Their garments and the large crucifixes hanging from their necks give away the fact that they are indeed nuns and not Muslim women, illustrating the irony of Nuttall's statement. Much like the debate that was sparked in Britain by the French face veil ban, UKIP's policy proposal prompted people to ask what such a ban in Britain would mean at a practical as well as ideological level. For example, the party was asked at a press conference whether such a ban would apply to beekeepers (Horton 2017). The cartoon shows how the act of veiling is not unique to the Muslim religion, and yet it is synonymous with Islam. Therefore, the mistake that Nuttall makes in the image is one that many members of the British public would also be likely to make.

Furthermore, Jennings also highlights how one can be considered 'more British' by virtue of being a Christian, depicting two Catholic nuns, one of whom is Caucasian and the other African-Caribbean. The image implies that by being a Christian nun, one has *chosen* to veil in such a manner, thereby affording nuns a permissibility to dress as such and to be honoured for doing so. In contrast, the Muslimah does not choose to wear the *burqa/niqab* and therefore should neither be allowed to wear nor respected for wearing such attire. Consequently, in the first scene Nuttall is enraged by the image of what he thinks are two veiled Muslim women walking down the street because he does not believe that veiling is compatible with 'Christian values.' When confronted by the confused nuns, he is rendered speechless in the second scene.

CONCLUSION

My examination of the portrayal of Muslim women sheds light on the way a community is made into an Other by using specific tropes as markers of difference in order to define what fits the definition of 'British' and what falls outside of it. Indeed, as we saw with the question of banning the face veil in Britain, the rebuttal to this was the fact that such a move fell outside what it means to be 'British,' bound up in ideas of tolerance. Ideas of embracing religious diversity as a positive value of the state have evolved from tolerating different interpretations of the Christian faith to a broader question of tolerating other faiths. My analysis of political cartoons exposes a prevailing yet problematic assumption that the act of veiling equates to a refusal of integration and acceptance of British values. The implication is that by wearing the *burqa/niqab*, the Muslimah—either of her own accord or at the behest of a controlling male figure—chooses invisibility, secrecy and withdrawal rather than visibility, forthrightness and participation in democratic society. If the Muslimah sees out, it is from a position of inscrutability, a privilege she is deemed not to deserve. She is, in effect, blind to the restrictiveness of her faith and the freedom of her country. The religious dimension of wearing the *burqa* is thus belittled and configured only as 'a self-conscious public statement' (Parekh 2006: 181). As Fernandez states:

> The gradual mutation of the veil from a symbol of religious identity to a contentious marker of difference paves the way for further contamination of the hijab as a sign of inequality, hostility to a democratic society, fundamentalism, as well as the blurred line between Islam and terror, breathing life into the savages-victims-saviours construct. (2009: 274)

The use of the term 'mutation' aptly denotes how the veil has undergone a transformation into a symbol that imputes negative messages, whereby the Muslim faith has little internal significance, and is defined only by its opposition to 'civilised' values.

Part of the resistance to accept the face veil may partly be explained by how it is frequently identified with the Taliban regime that governed Afghanistan from 1996 to 2001 (such as in Peter Brookes' 'New Jane Austen £10 Note [...]'). As such, it is frequently seen as a foreign practice imposed on women. This has had a major impact on how the *burqa/niqab* are used in images to highlight gender inequality and the oppression of women, even after the collapse of the Taliban regime. In this way, Islam is constructed as a system of primarily political ideals and goals, with the veil serving as evidence of Islamic subversion and resistance to Western culture. This follows Klug's theory that if 'antisemitism is the process of turning Jews into "Jews" then Islamophobia is the process of turning Muslims into "Muslims"' (Klug 2012: 678). The cartoons reflect contemporary concerns of terrorism originating from Muslim communities and regions. But those concerns become generalised and detached from specific contexts, with fear and suspicion becoming operative factors in how Muslims are portrayed. The *burqa/niqab* not only covers individuals; as a symbol read by non-Muslims it can serve to cloak particularities, covering all members of a religious group with a single stereotype.

Parekh points out that Muslims in Europe—like anyone else—have multifaceted identities, where gender, nationality and citizenship exist among multiple strands of identity. Thus, the term 'British Muslim' can mean a number of things—from denoting those who reside in the country without any patriotic sentiment to those who consider Britain their home and actively embrace 'British values.' Parekh emphasises the importance of how Muslims identify themselves to include words reflecting their citizenship or country of residence versus the simple, singular label 'Muslim.' This is because the latter homogenises Muslims and 'mould[s] them in their image of "true" Islam.' The danger is such that '[w]hen we refer to individuals and groups as Muslims *sans phrase*, we wittingly or unwittingly strip away or marginalise their other identities and walk into the Islamist trap' (Parekh 2006: 200). I find this marginalisation acutely present within cartoons, where a particular ideology of Islam is presented as dominant and overarching, thereby muting different discourses within the Muslim religion. Consequently, the cartoons perpetuate the image of the Muslimah as veiled, hidden and disembodied, ignoring not only the different aesthetics of veiling—from *hijab* to *burqa*—but the varied religious, cultural and personal motivations which these different forms might signify. On a deeper level, illustrations of the 'typical' Muslimah reflect the perception of Islam as monolithic, both theologically and socially. By this formula, the only ones who truly *see* Islam for what it is are, paradoxically, non-Muslims.

REFERENCES

Abbas, Tahir. (2008) 'Muslim Minorities in Britain: Integration, Multiculturalism and Radicalism in the Post-7/7 Period,' *Journal of Intercultural Studies*, 28(3), 287–300. https://doi.org/10.1080/07256860701429717

'Al-Qaeda in Yemen Claims Charlie Hebdo Attack.' (2015) *Al Jazeera*, 14 January. Available at: http://www.aljazeera.com/news/middleeast/2015/01/al-qaeda-yemen-charlie-hebdo-paris-attacks-201511410323361511.html [accessed 30 October 2017].

Alibhai-Brown, Yasmin. (2010) 'The Burka Empowering Women? You Must Be Mad, Minister,' *Daily Mail*, 21 July. Available at: http://www.dailymail.co.uk/debate/article-1296132/The-burka-empowering-women-You-mad-minister.html [accessed 22 February 2015].

'Blears Seeks to Reassure Muslims.' (2005) *BBC News*, 2 August. Available at: http://news.bbc.co.uk/1/hi/uk_politics/4736969.stm [accessed 30 October 2017].

Chrisafis, Angelique. (2009) 'Nicolas Sarkozy Says Islamic Veils Are Not Welcome in France,' *The Guardian*, 22 June. Available at: https://www.theguardian.com/world/2009/jun/22/islamic-veils-sarkozy-speech-france [accessed 30 October 2017].

ComRes. (2015) *Muslim Poll* [online]. Available at: http://www.comresglobal.com/wp-content/uploads/2015/02/BBC-Today-Programme_British-Muslims-Poll_FINAL-Tables_Feb2015.pdf [accessed 30 October 2017].

The Constitution of Afghanistan. (26 January 2004) Available at: http://www.afghanembassy.com.pl/afg/images/pliki/TheConstitution.pdf [accessed 30 Oct 2017].

Criado-Perez, Caroline. (2013) 'We Need Women on British Banknotes,' *Change.org*. Available at: https://www.change.org/p/we-need-women-on-british-banknotes [accessed 22 February 2015].

Curtis Jr., L. Perry. (1997) *Apes and Angels: The Irishman in Victorian Caricature*. Washington, DC: Smithsonian Institution Press.

Deedes, W. F. (2006) 'Muslims Can Never Conform to Our Ways,' *The Telegraph*, 20 October. Available at: http://www.telegraph.co.uk/comment/personal-view/3633349/Muslims-can-never-conform-to-our-ways.html [accessed 26 August 2018].

Dodd, Vikram. (2013) 'Burqa Fugitive Mohammed Ahmed Mohamed "Faced 20 Charges",' *The Guardian*, 8 November. Available at: http://www.theguardian.com/uk-news/2013/nov/08/*burqa*-fugitive-mohammed-ahmed-mohamed-20-charges [accessed 22 February 2015].

Elgot, Jessica. (2017) 'UKIP to Campaign to Ban Burqa and Sharia Courts, says Paul Nuttall,' *The Guardian*, 23 April. Available at: https://www.theguardian.com/politics/2017/apr/23/ukip-to-campaign-to-ban-burka-and-sharia-courts-says-paul-nuttall [accessed 30 October 2017].

The Employment Equality (Religion or Belief) Regulations 2003 [online]. Available at: http://www.legislation.gov.uk/uksi/2003/1660/contents/made [accessed 15 February 2015].

Fernandez, Sonya. (2009) 'The Crusade Over the Bodies of Women,' *Patterns of Prejudice*, 43(3–4), 269–286. https://doi.org/10.1080/00313220903109185

Foucault, Michel. (2008) 'Panopticism,' from *Discipline & Punish: The Birth of the Prison*, *Race/Ethnicity: Multidisciplinary Global Contexts*, 2(1), 1–12. Available at: https://www.jstor.org/stable/25594995 [accessed 26 August 2018].

Franks, Myfanwy. (2000) 'Crossing the Borders of Whiteness? White Muslim Women Who Wear the Hijab in Britain Today,' *Ethnic and Racial Studies*, 23, 917–929. https://doi.org/10.1080/01419870050110977

Hammer, Gili. (2016) '"If They're Going to Stare, at Least I'll Give Them a Good Reason To": Blind Women's Visibility, Invisibility, and Encounters with the Gaze,' *Signs: Journal of Women in Culture and Society*, 41(2), 409–432. Available at: https://www.journals.uchicago.edu/doi/pdfplus/10.1086/682924 [accessed 22 February 2015]. https://doi.org/10.1086/682924

Hennessy, Patrick. (2010) 'Burka Ban Ruled Out by Immigration Minister,' *Daily Telegraph*, 17 July. Available at: http://www.telegraph.co.uk/news/politics/7896751/Burka-ban-ruled-out-by-immigration-minister.html [accessed 22 February 2015].

Horton, Helena. (2017) '"What about Beekeepers?": UKIP mocked after being forced to clarify their veil-banning policy,' *Daily Telegraph*, 24 April. Available at: http://www.telegraph.co.uk/news/2017/04/24/beekeepers-ukip-mocked-forced-clarify-veil-banning-policy/ [accessed 30 October 2017].

'In Your Face.' (2011) *The Times*, 11 April, p. 2, *The Times Digital Archive*. Available at: http://find.galegroup.com/dvnw/infomark.do?&source=gale&prodId=DVN-W&userGroupName=kings&tabID=T003&docPage=article&docId=IF504210106&-type=multipage&contentSet=LTO&version=1.0 [accessed 26 August 2018].

'Jane Austen to be Face of The Bank of England £10 Note.' (2013) *BBC News*, 24 July. Available at: http://www.bbc.co.uk/news/business-23424289 [accessed 22 February 2015].

Klug, Brian. (2012) 'Islamophobia: A Concept Comes of Age,' *Ethnicities*, 12(5), 665–681. https://doi.org/10.1177/1468796812450363

Liberty. (n.d.) *Section 44 Terrorism Act* [online]. Available at: https://www.liberty-human-rights.org.uk/human-rights/justice-and-fair-trials/stop-and-search/section-44-terrorism-act [accessed 30 Oct 2017].

MCB (The Muslim Council of Britain's Research & Documentation Committee). (2015) *British Muslims in Numbers a Demographic, Socio-Economic and Health Profile of Muslims in Britain Drawing on the 2011 Census*. London: The Muslim Council of Britain. Available at: https://www.mcb.org.uk/wp-content/uploads/2015/02/MCBCensusReport_2015.pdf [accessed 18 August 2018].

Meer, N. and Modood, T. (2009) 'Refutations of Racism in the "Muslim Question",' *Patterns of Prejudice*, 43(3–4), 335–354. https://doi.org/10.1080/00313220903109250

Modood, Tariq. (2005) *Multicultural Politics: Racism, Ethnicity, and Muslims in Britain*. Minneapolis: University of Minnesota Press.

Modood, Tariq. (2006) 'British Muslims and the Politics of Multiculturalism,' in Modood, Tariq, Triandafyllidou, Anna and Zapata-Barrero, Ricard (eds.), *Multiculturalism, Muslims and Citizenship: A European Approach*. New York: Routledge, pp. 37–56.

Morrison, Karen. (2013) 'Muslim Woman Will Have to Remove Veil to Give Evidence,' *The Sun*, 16 September. Available at: https://www.thesun.co.uk/archives/news/1016924/muslim-woman-will-have-to-remove-veil-to-give-evidence/ [accessed 30 October 2017].

Murtagh, Peter. (1989) 'Rushdie in Hiding after Ayatollah's Death Threat,' *The Guardian*, 15 February. Available at: http://www.theguardian.com/books/1989/feb/15/salmanrushdie [accessed 22 February 2015].

NUS Black Students' Campaign. (2014) 'Birmingham Metropolitan College: Reverse Your Decision to Ban Muslim Students from Wearing Veils,' *Change.org*. Available at: https://www.change.org/p/birmingham-metropolitan-college-reverse-your-decision-to-ban-muslim-students-from-wearing-veils [accessed 22 February 2015].

Parekh, Bhikhu. (2006) 'Europe, Liberalism and the "Muslim Question",' in Modood, Tariq, Triandafyllidou, Anna and Zapata-Barrero, Ricard (eds.), *Multiculturalism, Muslims and Citizenship: a European Approach*. New York: Routledge, pp. 179–203.

Peachey, Kevin. (2013) 'Sir Winston Churchill to Feature on New Banknote', *BBC News*, 26 April. Available at: http://www.bbc.co.uk/news/business-22306707 [accessed 22 February 2015].

Prince, Rosa. (2010) 'Caroline Spelman: Wearing Burka Can Be "Empowering",' *Daily Telegraph*, 19 July. Available at: http://www.telegraph.co.uk/news/religion/7897848/Caroline-Spelman-wearing-burka-can-be-empowering.html [accessed 22 February 2015].

Qur'an: English Translation with Parallel Arabic text. (2010) Translated by M.A.S. Abdel Haleem. Oxford: Oxford University Press.

RAWA (Revolutionary Association of the Women of Afghanistan). (n.d.) *Some of the Restrictions Imposed by Taliban on Women in Afghanistan* [online]. Available at: http://www.rawa.org/rules.htm [accessed 30 October 2017].

Saul, Heather. (2013) 'Vince Cable Accuses Bank of England Officials of "Acting Like the Taliban",' *The Independent*, 24 July. Available at: http://www.independent.co.uk/news/business/news/vince-cable-accuses-bank-of-england-officials-of-acting-like-the-taliban-8729262.html [accessed 22 February 2015].

Seymour-Ure, Colin. (2001) 'What Future for the British Political Cartoon?' *Journalism Studies*, 2(3), 333–355. https://doi.org/10.1080/14616700120062202

Slack, James. (2010) 'Burkas Empower Women: Female Cabinet Minister Insists Freedom to Wear Muslim Veil is a Right,' *Daily Mail*, 20 July. Available at: http://www.dailymail.co.uk/news/article-1295665/Banning-burkas-UK-British-says-Green.html [accessed 22 February 2015].

The Terrorism Act 2000 (Remedial) Order 2011 [online]. Available at: https://www.legislation.gov.uk/uksi/2011/631/article/3/made [accessed 30 Oct 2017].

Yegenoglu, Meyda. (1998) 'Sartorial Fabric-Actions: The Enlightenment and Western Feminism,' in Yegenoglu, Meyda (ed.), *Colonial Fantasies: Towards a Feminist Reading of Orientalism*. Cambridge: Cambridge University Press, pp. 95–120. Available at: http://dx.doi.org/10.1017/CBO9780511583445.005 [accessed 22 February 2019]. https://doi.org/10.1017/CBO9780511583445.005

Tahnia Ahmed recently submitted her doctoral dissertation on 'Religious and Cultural Difference in Modern British Political Cartoons' at King's College London. She received her BA and MA from the University of Cambridge, and her MSt from the University of Oxford. Her previous publications include a chapter on the representation of British Sikhs in *Visualising a Sacred City: London, Art and Religion*, eds. Ben Quash, Chloe Reddaway and Aaron Rosen (I.B. Tauris, 2016). In addition to her academic work, Ahmed is a civil servant in the UK central government.

Chapter 3

Obscuring Two-Spirit Deaths in the Films *Conversion* and *Fire Song*

GABRIEL ESTRADA

Indigenous film historians interrogate the persistence of the 'disappearing Indian' trope across the Silent, Classic and Contemporary Hollywood eras. Documenting the ongoing struggles for Native American 'visual sovereignty,' or equitable Indigenous self-representation (Raheja 2011: 12), Raheja comments, 'Native American ghosts haunt the North American literary and visual cultural imagination simultaneously to remind settler nations of the unspeakable, horrific past and to commit representational genocide by writing contemporary Native American people out of the present and the future' (2011: 9). This ghostly dynamic remains common in contemporary slasher films such as *The Shining* (1980) by Jewish-American director Stanley Kubrick. These horror films set on Indigenous burial grounds evoke a distant settler colonial history of massacres rather than explore how contemporary Indigenous peoples confront genocidal historical trauma.

Marubbio interjects the importance of gendered bodies in the larger 'disappearing Indian' trope by highlighting the greater prevalence of Native American women's suicide in Hollywood film. The loss of the 'Indian Maiden's life in silent film serves to prevent both miscegenation and Indigenous futurity' (Marubbio 2006: 57). The US 1930 Film Production Code officially censored out positive miscegenation and queer romance film arcs. Classic cinema censors only allowed for interracial and queer relationships to appear on screen provided that the non-white or queer character committed suicide or died tragically. Waugh finds that Canadian national cinema had analogous moral restrictions on queer film images but these were more regionally controlled, especially in the metropolitan areas of 'Montreal, Toronto, and Vancouver' (2006: 12). The combined settler colonial and cis-heterosexist hegemonies of Hollywood are only overcome with the late 1980s' rise of AIDS gay/lesbian American Indian health videos (Estrada 2016: 399). It was at this time that the 1990 term 'two-spirit' was being formulated in Lesbian, Gay, Bisexual, Transgender and Queer (LGBTQ) Indigenous American circles in order to express male and female spirits in one body, to reclaim Indigenous-language third gender roles, and to transcend gender (Gilley 2014: 24). Moving beyond the 1900s' film stereotypes of ghostly 'Indians' and queer suicides, this chapter seeks to understand how post-millennial Indigenous North American directors obscure two-spirit-related deaths as a method of achieving visual sovereignty.

In viewing films from a Diné (Navajo) and Cree/Metis director, one finds different protocols surrounding the depiction of two-spirit-related death. Diné director Nanobah Becker incorporated a Diné prohibition against viewing a corpse in her 2006 film *Conversion* that critiques the impact of 1950s Christian proselytisation on the Navajo Nation. This ancient mortuary prohibition begins with the first two-spirit person created, following Diné protocol established after witnessing a dead two-spirit person engendered more deaths (Zolbrod 1987: 84–85). However, not all Indigenous directors share the prohibition against visualising death that some Diné do. Responding to 24% sexual assault rates among two-spirit/Indigenous transgender/gender non-conforming people (Grant, Motlett and Tanis 2011: 36) along with high rates of Indigenous youth suicide, Indigenous filmmakers grapple with conflicting cultural, spiritual and political protocols for showing violent murders, suicides and ghosts in two-spirit films. After analysing the death-avoidance of *Conversion*'s visual aesthetics, this essay considers the contrasting open suicide and ghost images in the 2015 feature film *Fire Song* by Cree/Metís/Danish director Adam Garnet Jones that follows a different set of cultural protocols as an Ontario-based Anishinaabe film. Like Becker, Jones avoids showing a culturally sensitive death; he foils the Classic Hollywood gay suicide trope when his two-spirit protagonist fails to kill himself. However, in creating a utopic two-spirit romantic resolution, Jones transfers some of the film's unresolved gendered violence onto the protagonist's ghostly ex-girlfriend who is imaged molested, jilted, raped and hanged.

CONVERSION (2006)

The nine-minute film *Conversion* directed and written by Becker uses a framework of anti-missionary themes to reclaim Diné linguistic, religious and visual protocols. The film is entirely spoken in the Diné language and subtitled in English, an act that resists the English-language Christian indoctrination that Becker's family experienced through US state-mandated boarding schools. The film begins with brief 1933 black-and-white footage of Diné family life in the traditional hogan, a log and earth-constructed house, and Diné chanters. The main story set in the 1950s is filmed in colour and centres on the mysterious death of a Diné grandfather and traditional healer immediately after a visit by aggressive Christian missionaries. In this narrative, the youngest granddaughter leads her aunt on a journey to explain the Christian intrusion. As part of depicting the earth-based belief system, *Conversion* honours Diné spiritual protocols by not showing the dead grandfather on screen, a protocol that began with the first Diné two-spirit death. Despite the aunt's warnings, the youngest granddaughter forms a strange fixation on a missionary image of Christ that she pieces together after her aunt has ripped it up. The short ends with the soundtrack of the 1933 chanters. This film analysis emphasises two key visual representations that Becker makes in *Conversion*: the first is a foregrounding of sacred matrilineal land and the second is an avoidance of visualising death.

In *Conversion*, the aunt arrives at a hogan to visit her ill father. He is asleep on sheepskins and surrounded by three of his grandchildren. Leaving the two grandsons in the hogan with their grandfather, the elder granddaughter steps outside and answers the aunt's repeated question in Diné. 'What happened?' is the English translation caption of the aunt's Diné spoken words. In Diné, the granddaughter responds, 'Some missionaries came here. They told Grampa to throw away his medicine bag. They said we don't listen to "God." Then Grampa left with them. When he came back, he laid down. He hasn't gotton up since.' The younger granddaughter, who had been wandering around outside the hogan, enters the shot and immediately leads the aunt on a long walk on open land to where the grandfather's medicine bag lies emptied on the ground. The aunt retrieves the empty bag from the ground, examines it, and then gathers it in her hand. Becker films this gathering moment in slow motion; it is the only slow motion part of the film. The empty pouch visually represents the loss of the grandfather's medicine traditions and it also foretells the loss of his life during the aunt's journey. This slow motion effect further correlates the coming of Christian missionaries with the loss of traditional medicine and health. While many Indigenous people keep core traditional spiritual practices as they adopt Christianity, this radical throwing away of all previous traditional medicines seems to represent an imbalance in the conversion process as it quickly leads to sickness. It is almost as if the grandfather is forced to commit spiritual and literal suicide by radically abandoning the medicine that will keep himself and his family in good health, 'peace' and 'harmony,' which some Diné link to the concept of 'hózhǫ́ (Werito 2014: 29). The slow motion could also indicate a thinking process on the aunt's part as she contemplates the colonial implications of the loss of medicine and the subsequent impact on 'hózhǫ́.

Upon returning from the journey with the grandfather's empty medicine bag, the aunt charges far ahead of the younger granddaughter and comes to a stop several metres from the hogan (**Figure 3.1**). A close-up shot of her face shows the strain of the grandfather's illness and the violation of Navajo traditional beliefs represented by the abandoned bag. The reverse shot in bright natural light is wide and encompasses a large foreground of desert sagebrush, the greens and tans of plants and grasses, and a taller juniper tree on the right of the hogan. Traditionally dressed in velvet blouses, calico dresses, woven belts, silver squash blossom necklaces with naja pendants, the women with their hair tied back in buns (*tsiiyééł*) with white yarn face each other, the elder granddaughter facing

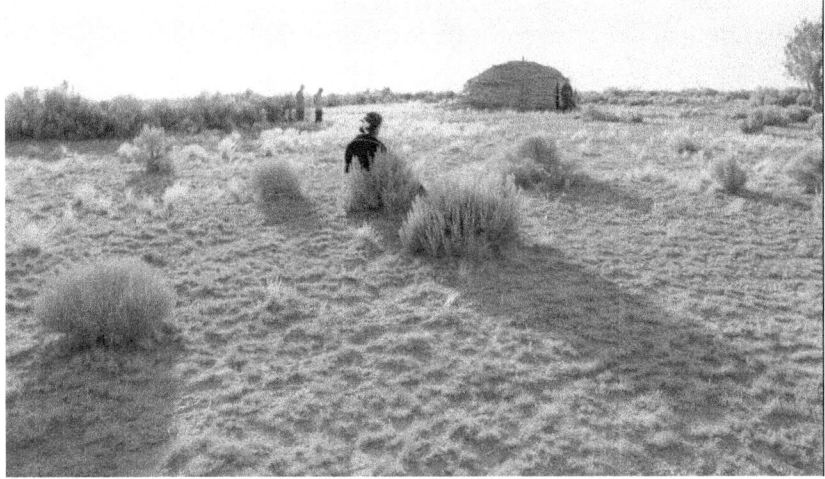

Figure 3.1 The respectful distance from death outside the hogan. *Conversion* (2006). Directed by Nanobah Becker. Park City, UT: Sundance Institute/Sundance Institute Native Initiative.

the camera in front of the hogan's blanketed door and the aunt looking away from the camera toward the hogan. Ominously, the two grandsons are now standing together outside, some yards to the left of the hogan, with their heads hanging down. 'It's too late,' announces the sad-faced granddaughter by the door. Immediately, the aunt's legs buckle and she falls to the ground in a seated position. The older granddaughter and two boys sit down by her and say nothing. The four together create a silent circle among the vast landscape of desert plants.

Figure 3.1 is one of many instances that indicate the overwhelming import that earth holds in Diné culture. This connection of spirituality and land was expressed in a film interview the author had with Becker in 2012:

> GE: What makes a Native filmmaker different than any other filmmaker? Is there anything visual that is different about any of the shots? ... Do you think there is anything particularly...Navajo...about the way you filmed?

> NB: One thing that...I feel like I make an effort to do in films that I direct and produce...is to include landscapes.... I worked with Blackhorse Lowe on his film...I helped produce *Shimasani*.... I said, 'we have to get Shiprock' because we were shooting out in that area.... It made the cut. We are on our ancestral homeland. The stories are in the land, in the landscape. So that's very important to me as an Indigenous filmmaker...and also trying to use the language.

Wide shots of earth as the Diné ancestral homeland dominate *Conversion*, as evidenced in the death scene filmed outside the traditional hogan. One notes that plants and landscape compose about four-fifths of the entire shot. This is an unusual ratio relative to Hollywood films that usually tightly restrict visualisations around individuals in their greatest moments of stress, such as the realisation of death. Becker filmed *Conversion* on the Navajo Nation, specifically the *Tzech'izhi Bito* (Ojo Encino) chequerboard area in New Mexico where her mother's clan is located. The deep matrilineal ties are indexed by the broad landscapes and use of the Diné language to show that relationship to land. Becker's clan sister provided the Diné dialogue in the film. All Diné clans derive from *'Asdzą́ą́ Nádleehé* or Changing Woman, the Mother Earth deity who created the Diné clans from her body (Begay 2014: 122). Becker traditionally identifies with the Diné matrilineal clans of her four grandparents. She is of the *Kin łichii'nii* (Red House) clan and born for the *Bilagáana* (Euro-American) clan. Her maternal grandfather is of the *Todich'ii'nii* (Bitter Water) clan and her paternal grandfather is of the *Bilagáana* clan. Despite having a Euro-American father and being raised in Los Angeles, Becker found ways to strengthen connections with her mother's Diné land, language, and clan throughout the filming process.

When Becker states that she made *Conversion* for a primarily Diné audience, she not only refers to nationalistic feeling common within many nations, she also intimates a specific Diné sense of earth. Diné oral traditions confirm that the current earth surface is but the last for the Diné to inhabit. *Diné Bahane'* (The People's Story) recounts the three migrations of the Diné from the original first world and their emergence into the present fourth world. Each emergence begins as the Diné reach a hole in the sky of the lower world and move through it and onto the surface of the next one just above the last world (Begay 2014: 121). The lessons of life on the surface of the present world resonate with all the lessons learned in the previous three worlds below. The origin of Diné death and ghost protocols involve the two-spirit figure of the *nádleeh* (changing one) twins, who were intersex or genderqueer, 'neither entirely male nor entirely female' (Zolbrod 1987: 51). The extraordinary twin *nádleeh* were the first children of First Woman and First Man. Zolbrod recounts that after the emergence of the Diné from the third to the fourth and present world, one of the *nádleeh* stopped breathing and disappeared when laid out to rest. Two Diné men who saw the dead *nádleeh* down through the emergence hole to the third world below also died within four days. To this day, Diné traditionalists, whose ancestral beliefs have a significant place in their practices, often avoid seeing the dead.

The Diné consequences of not letting the dead go are explored in *Two Spirits*, a documentary about the hate killing of the *nádleeh* youth Fred Martinez. *Diné Bizaad* (Navajo language) teacher Dr Wesley Thomas narrates the beginning of the *Two Spirits* film in which he recalls the Diné emergence from the black world, to the blue world, to the yellow world, to the present world of many colours. Thomas also explains a Diné sense that the deceased has four days to depart to the next world, to go back to the beginning, and that in this mourning period not even the deceased's name is to be mentioned. When Fred's mother does not accept her child's departure as a result of a bloody hate crime, the spirit of Fred returns to haunt her trailer and dreams. In the film, the mother is somewhat surprised to find that her attachment has delayed Fred from moving on to the spirit world. She has a ceremony to release Fred's spirit, but she also sits at the site of his murder and prays for him, which is a Christian-influenced practice now more common with widespread Diné conversion (Shepardson 1978: 385).

The shot in **Figure 3.1** is a prime example of Becker's respect for Diné spiritual mortuary protocols learned long ago between worlds, the lessons that Thomas recalls in *Two Spirits*. Becker explains, 'Navajos have a lot of taboos' (2012), adding, 'I had to make some changes in my script in regards to cultural sensitivity surrounding death and Navajo beliefs' (Guerresio 2012). Originally, Becker showed the corpse of the dead grandfather in the hogan but then removed the image at the request of Diné audiences when she first screened the film on Navajo Nation. Becker edited the images to affirm a Diné audience's sense that a body after death should not be seen, even on film. By keeping the realisation of death so far from the hogan, Becker respects the sense of space that the dead body can occupy in Diné culture. As Thomas indicated, this honouring of the dead's space extends even to not mentioning the dead person's name within the four days after death. It may be for this reason that the granddaughter merely says, 'It's too late' rather than call her 'Grampa' by his relational name as she does while he is still living.

While the link between *Conversion*'s visual death avoidance and two-spirit/Indigenous LGBTQ people is not obvious, such a link becomes possible if one considers the origins of the Diné death protocols and the history of emergence. That Becker edited out the grandfather's dead body from her film subtly references part of the legacy of the *nádleeh* within Diné culture, a mortuary protocol established many times over in Diné experiences. This initial *Conversion* analysis does not focus on queer characters; however it does queer the historical, cinematic and cultural context of *Conversion*. To mention this ancient *nádleeh* connection resists contemporary Christian Diné narratives that completely deny any use for *nádleeh* existence in Diné history and contemporary times (Estrada 2011: 172). While the first *nádleeh* had a part in establishing death protocols, a more celebrated *nádleeh* role is to bring balance between genders. Transgender Diné director Sydney Freeland created the feature *Drunktown's Finest* (2015) to educate her community about the integral place of the *nádleeh* within Diné traditions. In her film, the grandfather explains the term *nádleeh* to his transgender granddaughter and retells the story of how the *nádleeh* brought balance back to the Diné by helping resolve a dispute between men and women who had separated across a river. Due to the influence of settler colonial cis-heterosexist Christianity, however, this idea of gender balance both within the *nádleeh* body and between men and women of the same community is highly suppressed among many Diné. These gender understandings are only making a limited comeback with community activism, education, and films like *Two Spirits* and *Drunktown's Finest*. The coming of Christianity in *Conversion* foretells a change in the gender balance as the US government implements policies that weaken Diné women's central place in society as well as virtually banishing the acknowledgement of *nádleeh* roles. Denetdale accounts for the ways in which settler colonial cis-heteropatriarchy becomes nationalised in contemporary Diné governance as being merely 'traditional' instead of colonial (2006: 10). *Conversion* reinstates Diné women as central to society and only Diné females speak in the film. Although the film's Christian conversion is framed in a heterosexist settler colonial context, it is still the female casts' choice to reject or consider the missionary option despite the ongoing violence implied by the grandfather's death.

The figure of Christ on Diné land enters the film's final scenes as a complicated sign of hyper-masculine settler colonial conquest. When the aunt rips up the missionary leaflet and admonishes in Navajo, 'This is not ours. Not for us. Not for you,' the younger granddaughter surreptitiously gathers the three parts of the shredded image and quickly steals away alone to a distant outcropping of rock to gaze at Jesus until dusk. The final film image shows the girl's small silhouette hunched over the Jesus image against the yellow sunset in the west. The implications of this final image are many. Is the granddaughter the convert to which the title *Conversion* alludes? Will she lose her Diné language as Becker's mother did at a Christian boarding school? While this is a future possibility, the melding of her body's outline and the surrounding rock indicates her connection to 'Asdząą Nádleehé (Changing Woman) and Diné spirituality. The youngest granddaughter remains rooted in her land and culture in the final shot as the 1933 chanting of a Diné social dance returns with the darkening of this last image. By ending her film with Diné chanting, Becker indicates the resilience of Diné medicine, land relations, language and culture. Even after her family's loss of traditional Diné language and chanting, the singing eventually returned to the family in the generation after hers (Estrada 2014: 528). Thus, even if the girl converts to Christianity and suffers cultural loss, the repetition of the 1933 chanting promises a way back to land and matrilineal clans within Navajo Nation.

Contemporary films like *Conversion* only begin to make up for the century of settler colonial images that dissolved Diné spiritual protocol into hyper-masculine images of settler colonial conquest. In a context of hegemonic Hollywood images, Becker's choice to limit death and ghost images is noteworthy. While many Hollywood Westerns, such as *The Searchers* (1956), thrived on the spectre of violent cowboy and Indians deaths filmed on Navajo Nation, *Conversion*'s camera keeps a respectful distance and silence where the dead are concerned. And, in contrast to *The Shining* in which the settler colonial protagonist hurls a tennis ball against the large painted representations of the Diné Holy People as a symbolic assault on Indigenous religion, Becker emphasises a Diné sense of maintaining a balanced life on earth even in the most difficult situations involving the lethal missionary intrusion into Diné culture. Becker's reclaiming of Diné language and spiritual protocols shows a willingness to counter both secular and religious colonisation that the US continues to impose upon Navajo Nation. With an honouring of Diné death protocols, language and matrilineal landscapes, the urban and partly Euro-American Becker contributes to the struggle for Diné visual sovereignty. This final emphasis on sovereignty is to remind readers that *Conversion* is not an English-language US film; its themes, language and visual styles reflect important aspects of an emerging Diné national cinema. A full citizen of Navajo Nation, Becker is already noted for her contributions to Diné national film (Lewis 2012: 173).

FIRE SONG (2015)

Fire Song's depiction of suicide and sexual assault engages scholarly debates on the potential impact of viewing graphic violence. For example, Cárdenas interrogates 'the spread of affect such as shock, grief and numbness,' which result from an uncritical 'incitement' to media visibility of racialised and transgender violence (2017: 169). Diné-themed films demonstrate a diversity of perspectives on the issue of viewing disturbing images. In contrast with the no-corpse Diné visual protocol that Becker respected, *Two Spirits* by Euro-American Lydia Nibley re-enacts the murder of the Diné *nádleeh* youth Fred Martinez by including graphic scenes of Fred's bloody stoning and quick shots of his post-mortem body. Clearly Nibley's shocking images were meant to elicit outrage against the hate crime, especially when framed by the crying narratives of Fred's mother who fought hard to bring Fred's killer to justice. In their review of *Two Spirits*, Knabe and Pearson praise Nibley for attacking the cis-heterosexist settler colonialism that motivated Fred's homicide; however, they also note how the film's 'partial re-enactment of the murder...runs the risk of re-traumatizing its audience, whether LGBT or straight, Indigenous or non-Indigenous' (Knabe and Pearson 2013: 388). On one hand, to not portray the two-spirit/LGBTQI murder is to run the risk that audiences will fail to act politically without the stimulus of violent imagery. Others like Cárdenas respond that shock tactics compromise the mental health of vulnerable audiences. In addition, directors who focus solely on Indigenous cultural dysfunctions and violence inevitably face charges that they are merely reinforcing stereotypes of tragic indigeneity.

Adam Garnet Jones is a queer Cree/Metís/Danish film director who models visual sovereignty and two-spirit activism in his 2015 film *Fire Song* that features an all-Indigenous cast. As writer and director, Jones complicates gay 'coming out' film tropes by requiring his queer Anishinaabe protagonist Shane (Andrew Martin, Mohawk) to deal with multiple Indigenous social problems in the following plot. After Shane's sister commits suicide, Shane faces the choice to stay on the homophobic Ontario reserve as a support for his mourning mother Jackie (Jennifer Podemski, Anishinaabe/Leni Lenape/Metís) or to leave for the university and queer freedoms of Toronto with his reserve boyfriend David (Harley Legarde-Beacham, Ojibway). As the plot advances, Shane must also extract himself from the local reserve drug trade and from being implicated in the suicide of his ex-girlfriend Tara (Mary Galloway, Cowinchan) who suffers heartbreak, incest, alcoholism and rape before hanging herself. As Shane evades police who wrongfully suspect him in Tara's rape, David prevents Shane from killing himself in a climactic scene at a lake. With the evolving support of their respective families, David and Shane openly share their plan to move to Toronto together as a couple. As Shane's mother finally releases her daughter's ghost by ceremonially burning the daughter's old possessions, she tells Shane she fully supports his move.

The scenes of Tara's suicide and Shane's failed suicide are central in this analysis. First, a drunk Tara witnesses Shane kissing David in the night. When Tara confronts Shane about the kiss, Shane will not respond to her under pressure from David who does not want to be outed as gay. While David and Shane abandon Tara to solidify their plans to move to Toronto, the heartbroken Tara rushes off, correctly ascertaining Shane's sexual preference for other men and the sham of their own plans to move to the big city. At an abandoned house, Tara finds comfort in the arms of the homophobic Kyle (Brendt Thomas Diabo, Mohawk) who proceeds to sexually assault her, despite her active resistance. While Jones does not picture the actual penetration, he does show the beginning of the sexual assault and includes Tara's screams from afar as the rape begins. When Tara awakens early in the morning she cries as she finds herself abandoned and half-nude on an old mattress. Inside the gutted house, she approaches the place where she will hang herself and considers the wires that hang down from the wooden frame.

After a contrasting cut to yellow wildflowers, the spirit of Tara kisses the still-sleeping Shane in his bed. As Tara's lips leave Shane's cheek, the resulting space reveals a sun flare from the window, a bright sign indicating that Tara's spirit has left her earthly pain. She is not returning as a vengeful spirit to curse Shane for abandoning her in darkness, but rather as one who has love, light and hope for his future. The suicide ghost of Shane's sister also constantly roams the house and most often is visualised as a comforting spirit by the side of her mourning mother. In contrast to Diné culture, the Anishinaabe cultural context of *Fire Song* better allows for the benevolent suicide ghosts to visually remain near Shane and family until they are released and acknowledged later in the film.

Upon awaking, Shane goes to search for Tara, first at her house, shadowed by Tara's father's alcoholic and incestuous advances on Tara, and then at the abandoned house where Shane once evaded Tara's sexual advances and where the rape occurred. The first fade to black falls as Shane enters the empty door frame of the dark abandoned house. Because the interior of the gutted house is heavily shadowed, sharp sounds gain prominence and add to the sense of disorientation and loss. Against the diegetic chatter of birds is a strange sound of swooping wind, like a sword or a body swinging through air. A soundtrack bass drum pulses the moment Shane enters the house and the next two-second fade to black occurs. Shane reappears inside the house and kicks one of the many old bottles that litter the ground as the soundtrack intensifies with long digital baritone notes and the eerie sound of crinkling. The ominous swooping sound occurs a second time before a third two-second fade to black. After a cut back to the house, the black outline of Shane is visible walking slowly forward through the wooden studs of the house. The audience can hear his diegetic expiration and the ominous music remains intense. The swooping sound reoccurs within the fourth two-second fade to black. In the last cut to the house, the intense eerie soundtrack intensifies with a mechanical high-pitched vibrato sound. Again, Shane's exhalation is audible. A shadowy Shane turns to confront Tara's body hanging from the wiring of the wooden house frame. The camera refocuses to clearly show her hanged body facing the camera and outlined against the sunny window. 'No! No! Nooo! Tara!' screams Shane as the final fade to black mechanically descends without pity.

While this last fade to black clearly represents the tragedy of Tara's suicide, the earlier four fade to blacks are meant to prepare the audience for the final dark suicide revelation. The film's reliance on the colour black as symbol for sunset, night, and the ending of light and life finds resonance in both popular and Anishinaabe understandings of colour. Westernised audiences will recognise the deathly connotations of black as an indication of funerals and mourning. From a traditionalist perspective, however, Anishinaabe elder Lillian Pitawanakwat explains black as representing the west or *epangishmok* side of the medicine wheel that incorporates meanings of sunset or 'death of the day,' fall, adulthood and heartfelt evaluation. She retells the Anishinaabe story of the strawberry in relation to the black direction in which adults develop emotional maturity, in part by confronting the full implications of the death of loved ones, even the unintentional killing of one's own brother (Pitawanakwat 2006). While Shane is not to blame for Tara's death, he did abandon her, which left her more vulnerable to the sexualised dangers of her reserve. Like the older brother in the ancient Anishinaabe strawberry story, Shane must deal with issues of guilt and acceptance regarding his unintentional role in the tragic death of a girl he loved.

The director related his take on visualising Tara's suicide and Shane's suicide attempt as deeply personal. Jones reports that he himself considered suicide through much of his youth, but was saved by participation in 'queer youth circles,' and artistic outlets which led to Indigenous filmmaking (Sanchez 2016). Growing up in urban Edmonton and later moving to the Ontario capital Toronto, Jones notes that the larger youth suicide motif of the film also came from the stories of youth suicide told by people he met from reserves (Canadian Press 2015). In responding to critiques that the film is overburdened with issues, Jones acknowledges that youth suicide is often multiply motivated. 'There's no easy answer, there's complexity, and Shane has options,' he concludes (Pecore 2016). I would counter Jones' own assessment of complication in his film by outlining how Tara's rape appears to operate as a transfer of the feature's gendered violence from the male two-spirit body onto the First Nation female body.

Tara's hanged body indicates a kind of heterosexual sacrifice for the success of the two-spirit romance in the film; the straight rival Tara must die so that the Shane and David can subsequently consummate their two-spirit relationship in the zero-sum game logic of the film. While the film could have examined Tara's death as emblematic of the high rates of femicide on reserves, a dynamic dramatised in the 2017 *Wind River* by Euro-American Taylor Sheridan, Tara's molestation, rape and suicide are displaced in the two-spirit romantic trajectory of the film. Subsequent scenes show the quick police capture of the rapist Kyle, and his drug-selling crew, in an immediate resolution to the true crime aspect of the film. Million would problematise Kyle's police arrest by voicing concerns that Western-model legal systems lack Indigenous rehabilitation (2013: 38). More importantly, neither Tara's incestuous father nor Shane systematically work through Tara's loss. In addition, *Fire Song* does not explore either the settler colonial historical trauma upon which high rates of violence towards Indigenous women are predicated, such as the systematic sexual abuse that dominated Indian residential school programmes of the late 1800s to the mid-1900s. These and other historical forces could illuminate why Tara's father and male peer sexually assault her. Other aspects of settler colonial trauma might better explain why poverty is rampant on the reserve. Audiences do not leave the theatre understanding how Anishinnaabe perpetrators and victims of sexual abuse are successfully organising themselves to heal sexual violence on reserves through traditional Anishinaabe ways of knowing and being (Gross 2014: 236). Although the film does show Shane attending an Indigenous programme on the reserve to help prevent suicide and to support a community grieving process in response to Tara's death, the programme never mentions ways to recover from or prevent sexual assault and rape, the two immediate causes of Tara's suicide. In terms of Indigenous feminist health care, the treatment of Tara's rape is problematic.

To have Tara's female body veil two-spirit oppression lessens the healing potential of the film that made explorations into two-spirit intersectional violence. If Shane outwardly showed his femininity as he momentarily does while being spooned or held by David, who only sometimes passes as heterosexual, the implication is that Shane might also be raped, sexually assaulted, jilted and abandoned. With this insight, Shane shouts 'No! No! Nooo!' upon seeing Tara's body not only for the loss of his girlfriend, but also for the death of his heterosexuality and masculine privilege as her suicide plunges him deeper into publicly identifying as a two-spirit person of more ambivalent gender and sexuality.

Tara's hanged corpse partially operates to transfer the anti-feminine violence from Shane's body that passes as masculine and heterosexual onto that of Tara. The lack of parallel gendered assault against the two-spirit characters is worth reconsidering in light of other two-spirit films. After all, two-spirit people experience high rates of sexual assault, addiction, gendered bullying, abandonment and suicide. For example, Karina Walters (Choctaw) notes that '49%' of her lesbian/gay/two-spirit/bisexual Honor Project cohort 'reported they had been raped or sexually assaulted,' highlighting the need to better understand two-spirit mental health and substance abuse challenges that correlate with high levels of several bias-related victimisations (Parker, Duran and Walters 2017: 71).

In *Deep Inside Clint Star* (1999), Dene-descendent Clint Star/Alberta alternately interviews, cajoles, ignores and harasses his Indigenous interviewees about their intimate experiences of rape, suicide, sexual abuse, queer sexuality and death. Star killed himself only three years after completing this 1999 Gemini Award-winning film, further dramatising the high impact of suicide among queer, poor and Indigenous people. When Star filmed parts of gay interviews in grainy black and white, he was representing the unresolved poverty and grittiness of sexualised violence that *Fire Song* avoids in its homonormative, relatively hopeful ending that is also beautifully filmed.

Deep Inside Clint offers important contrasts in female resilience and the vulnerability of the male two-spirit body that *Fire Song* masks through Tara's eroticised and abused body. For example, when Star interviews the Indigenous Tawny Mane in a seedy hotel room about her experiences with drinking and sexual violence, she recalls a trajectory of survival and change.

> Clint Star: Maggie why did you stop drinking?
> Tawny Mane: I used to get in trouble when I drank. I got really wasted into unconsciousness. These three other guys at the party raped me.
> Clint Star: That sucks.
> Tawny Mane: I just went on with life. I never drink anymore.
> Clint Star: You're the best. You kick ass.

Unlike the reserve-bound Tara, the urban adoptee Tawny Mane stops drinking and 'moves on' from the rape, though not without serious doubts. Her narrative would have provided balance to *Fire Song* that prominently features the suicides of Shane's younger sister and ex-girlfriend. Because Tara's rape and immanent suicide potentially trigger the traumatic experiences of audience members who survive sexual assault, a female survivor who works through part of her sexual trauma could help some audiences better resolve their own issues. *Fire Song* could also use more settler colonial historical background to explain the colonial source of modern Indigenous gendered violence. In contrast with *Fire Song*'s absent history, the two-spirit film *My Own Private Lower Post* (2008) by Teslin Tlingit councilperson Duane Gastant' Aucoin is very careful to trace the alcoholic domestic violence his mother suffered back to her gendered abuse in the state-mandated Indian residential schools. Walters confirms that two-spirit/Indigenous LGBTQ people show higher rates of 'suicidality, alcohol problems, and drug use if they have boarding school experience,' (Parker, Duran and Walters 2017: 68)—conditions that, Aucoin confirms, can especially impact the next generation as historical trauma if there are no sustained communal and healing interventions.

That Star quickly manoeuvres around the serious subject of alcoholism and sexual assault with supportive but almost knee-jerk statements regarding Tawny Mane's rape resonates with his reticence to explore his own sexual trauma. The porn-inspired title *Deep Inside Clint Star* indicates that Star is penetrable in his male body. Yet, while constantly posing in erotic modes and demanding that an establishing shot centre on his own 'ass,' Star only later admits that he never has sex. When he initially shares, 'When I was a kid my uncle was a pedophile...there was sex all through the family...it was weird...,' the audience gains the only 'deep' insight into what motivates the feature's fixation on sexual vulnerability in a film in which no one has sex. It appears in part that Star wishes to heal from his own queer molestation but is too afraid to overcome this fear by actually showing mutually satisfying sex, queer or otherwise.

Despite the hopeful trajectory of the two-spirit protagonists, *Fire Song* has its own related fear of homoeroticism and censorship. While Tara and Shane are shown deep kissing and dry humping in their underwear as they initiate Shane's loss of virginity, David and Shane only hold or hug each other when clothed (**Figure 3.2**). They never kiss or begin copulation as Shane and Tara do. That Jones offers only veiled hints of two-spirit erotic satisfaction bows to heteronormative standards, including shooting Tara's young female body as the object of the heterosexual male gaze. David's

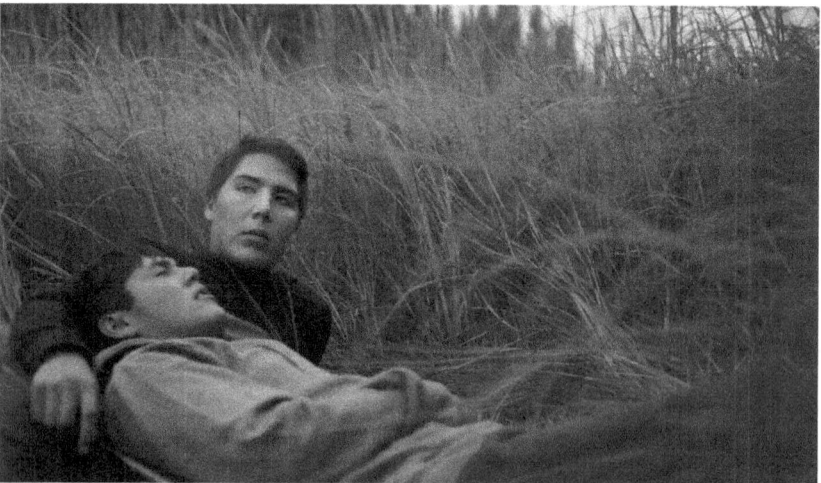

Figure 3.2 David holds Shane by the rice fields. *Fire Song* (2015). Directed by Adam Garnet Jones. Toronto: Big Soul Productions.

quip that he doesn't 'have sex with little boys' is a throw-away indication of deeper fears of homoeroticism that the film eclipses with clear shots of Tara's female body. The absence of male-bodied two-spirit sex across decades points to a persistent self-censorship on the part two-spirit directors. Dimas reminds us that queer Indigenous intergenerational trauma requires healing at all physical, emotional, mental, erotic and spiritual levels (2017: 79). The censorship of two-spirit erotic images needs resolution in subsequent films.

Tara's suicide ultimately drives Shane to attempt to take his own life. He struggles with survivor's guilt in relation to two intimate suicides. To add insult to injury, he is blamed for Tara's rape and becomes a fugitive from the law. In desperation, Shane realises that he has no real options to pay for his mother's leaky roof even after working odd jobs, harvesting wild rice, and selling drugs on the reserve. After a failed late-night attempt to steal money from a drug-dealer, Shane and David only manage to steal twenty dollars and a gun which Shane takes to the shadowy edge of the lake. Full of loss and frustration, Shane shouts at David, 'I'm poisonous—fucking poisonous—to everyone!' before blindly charging into the rippling lake with the gun. The soundtrack surges with the same high-pitched sound and booming drum that sounded at Tara's hanging to signal another impending suicide. Shane stares down the muzzle of the gun and begins to press it against his temple. David ignores Shane's commands to 'Just go! Go! Go!' and tackles Shane in the lake, holding him underwater until Shane loses hold of the gun and the suicidal intent subsides. Both young men are dressed in black which augments the dark visual theme as a representation of the loss of life. They climb back to shore dripping wet and glare at the disturbed lake. After a sober moment, they hug each other in solace. Here, *Fire Song*'s audiences benefit from the rare sight of a two-spirit youth saving the life of his own boyfriend. This refusal to depict yet another suicide in the film is meant to emphasise the strength of two-spirit lovers to survive the multiple tragedies that occur on Anishinaabe Ontario and Canadian reserves. As with Becker, not visualising death is a key statement of cultural values and respect for life.

Fire Song partially masks both historical two-spirit roles and the historical trauma of Christianity. For example, Christian residential schools especially erased the memory of Indigenous multigendered systems. In resistance to settler colonial cis-heteropatriarchy, the six-minute *Two Spirited* (2007) by Cree director Sharon Desjarlais documents the integral roles that two-spirit people historically enjoyed among the Stoney Nakoda. That Desjarlais highlights an Indigenous elder interviewee recounting this two-spirit history is important given the respect that oral traditions and elders often have in traditional Indigenous societies (Estrada 2010: 110–111). Knowledge of two-spirit history supports the short's arguments for a healthy two-spirit presence amongst today's Indigenous Nations. After years of struggle, the Nakoda protagonist Geeyo reclaims a pow-wow spot as a male-bodied two-spirit jingle-dress dancer, a category almost always reserved for female-bodied dancers. In contrast to the informed elder of *Two Spirited*, *Fire Song*'s traditionalist grandmother Evie, played by two-spirit activist Chacaby (Ojibwa-Cree), actually makes strong intimations against David's two-spirit desires. Ironically, in her own autobiography Chacaby shows clear education on two-spirit traditions, writing, 'two-spirit, same-sex couples used to play an important role in Anishinaabe communities...[and] were once loved and respected' (2016: 65). By shrouding two-spirit historical roles and settler colonial trauma, Jones limits important aspects of healing that many two-spirit and Indigenous leaders report as integral aspects of lessening contemporary gendered violence (Million 2013: 91). In short, *Fire Song* is unclear about traditional support for two-spirit people. Because of this, it cannot explain the settler colonial impact of the cis-heterosexist Christian Church to give a context for the graphic gendered violence that Indigenous people do to each other and to themselves throughout the film.

Fire Song's final resolution of multiple issues is abrupt, perhaps motivated by homonormative and Indigenous activist needs to show quick resolutions of queer Indigenous issues. When Shane and David wake up together in David's room, where they slept for the night, David's grandmother Evie and David's dysfunctional mother surprise them both by making breakfast. Not only do they allow David and Shane to sit with them as an acknowledged couple for the first time, they also explain their plan to sell the mother's home and live together in the grandmother's home. The two women have had a chat in which Shane's mother shared that a medicine person predicted Shane's two-spirit nature from birth, a narrative that Evie absorbs without comment. The mother's decision to sell the house and live with Evie frees Shane from the responsibility of fixing the roof and makes his future with David in Toronto a supported reality.

Although initially homophobic, Evie blesses David and Shane's hands and foreheads with kisses in the film's finale. This scene shows the four standing before the piled-up belongings from Shane's dead sister that are meant to be burnt to release her spirit. This is a surprise as the mother had fiercely held on to all her belongings in her intense mourning throughout most of the movie. 'You know, my son,' affirms the mother as the flames

Shane has lit begin to consume the deceased's boxes of memories, 'You can do anything. You can.' This is the emotional evolution that the mother long refused while mourning and it enables Shane to leave without feeling filial guilt. Set in the late afternoon, this final ceremonial burning marks the greatest resistance to being left emotionally submerged in the darkness of suicide and grief. The bright fire represents Shane's decision to live rather than shoot himself and it lights the way for Shane's ultimate success in moving with David to Toronto, with its utopic prospects of education, jobs and queer-friendly social spaces. Despite some gender limitations, *Fire Song*'s dedication to an all-Indigenous cast, queer youth and visual sovereignty make it an important addition to two-spirit and Indigenous youth suicide film. Added to US Netflix in 2017 and removed in 2019, *Fire Song* is now one of the most viewed two-spirit films in recent times. Audiences will likely agree that the ambitious *Fire Song* provides broad support for two-spirit youth in multiply dire situations.

CONCLUSION

Both Becker and Jones take care in how they visualise death. Becker accomplishes an important feat in responding to the visual protocols that her Diné audience imparted to her. By refusing to show a corpse on-screen, Becker acknowledges a respect for Diné culture that stems from the original two-spirit death as passed down through multiple oral traditions. While Becker is conservative in visualising corpses due to her matrilineal Diné cultural protocols, the Cree/Metís Jones is more free to depict spirits and even suicide in his queer youth suicide-themed film. In the ambitious film *Fire Song*, Jones uses visual sovereignty to show the strength of two-spirit survivors to deal with great losses surrounding issues of homophobia, youth suicides, sexual assault, drug trade/addiction and poverty. He refuses to offer the heteronormative queer suicide images common in Hollywood history. However, his graphic depiction of Tara's hanged body as the sacrificial heterosexual femme body cloaks gendered violence against two-spirit people. Of the two films, Becker's film better contextualises settler colonial gendered and religious violence. While *Fire Song* may inspire some audiences to better support two-spirit people and suicidal Indigenous youth, its strong images may re-traumatise other audiences. Nonetheless, through differing visualisations of suicide, mortality and violence, both Becker and Jones make important gains in visualising sovereignty by obscuring key deaths in their gendered and two-spirit films.

FILMOGRAPHY

Conversion. (2006) Directed by Nanobah Becker. Park City, UT: Sundance Institute/Sundance Institute Native Initiative.
Deep Inside Clint Star. (1999) Directed by Clint Alberta. Toronto: National Film Board of Canada.
Drunktown's Finest. (2015) Directed by Sydney Freeland. Tulsa: Indion Entertainment Group.
Fire Song. (2015) Directed by Adam Garnet Jones. Toronto: Big Soul Productions.
My Own Private Lower Post. (2008) Directed by Duane Gastant' Aucoin. Teslin, Yukon: DGA Productions and T'senaglobe Media.
Two Spirited: First Stories. (2007) Directed by Sharon Desjarlais. Toronto: National Film Board of Canada.
The Shining. (1980) Directed by Stanley Kubrick. Los Angeles: Warner Brothers.
Two Spirits. (2010) Directed by Lydia Nibley. Los Angeles: Say Yes Quickly Productions.
Wind River. (2017) Directed by Taylor Sheridan. Marksville, LA: Acadia Entertainment Production.

REFERENCES

Becker, Nanobah. (2012) Personal interview with author.
Begay, Yolynda. (2014) 'Historic and Demographic Changes that Impact the Future of the Diné and the Development of Community-Based Policy,' in Lee, Lloyd L. (ed.), *Diné Perspectives: Revitalizing and Reclaiming Navajo Thought*. Tucson: University of Arizona Press, pp. 105–128.
The Canadian Press. (2015) 'Profile: Adam Garnet Jones: Fire Song,' *The Canadian Press.* Available at: https://www.ctvnews.ca/entertainment/tiff-film-profile-adam-garnet-jones-fire-song-1.2561956 [accessed on 26 February 2019].
Cárdenas, Micha. (2017) 'Dark Shimmers: The Rhythm of Necropolitical Affect in Digital Media,' in Gosset, Reina, Stanley, Eric A. and Burton, Johanna (eds.), *Trap Door: Trans Cultural Production and the Politics of Visibility*. Cambridge: Massachusetts Institute of Technology Press, pp. 161–182.
Chacaby, Ma-Nee with Plummer, Mary Louisa. (2016) *A Two-Spirit Journey: The Autobiography of a Lesbian Ojibwa-Cree Elder*. Winnipeg: University of Manitoba Press.
Denetdale, Jennifer Nez. (2006) 'Chairmen, Presidents, and Princesses: The Navajo Nation, Gender, and the Politics of Tradition,' *Wicazo Sa Review*, 21(1), 9–28.
Dimas, Bernice. (2017) 'Queeranderismo,' in Facio, Elisa and Lara, Irene (eds.), *Fleshing the Spirit: Spirituality and Activism in Chicana, Latina, and Indigenous Women's Lives*. Tucson: University of Arizona Press, pp. 76–80.
Estrada, Gabriel S. (2010) 'Two-Spirit Film Criticism: Fancydancing with Imitates Dog, Desjarlais, and Alexie,' *Post Script: Essays in Film and the Humanities*, 29(3), 106–118.
Estrada, Gabriel S. (2011) 'Two Spirits, Nádleeh, and LGBTQ Navajo Film,' *American Indian Culture and Research Journal*, 35(4), 167–190.

Estrada, Gabriel S. (2014) 'Navajo Sci-Fi Film: Matriarchal Visual Sovereignty in Nanobah Becker's *The 6th World*,' *Journal of the American Academy of Religion*, 82(2), 521–530.

Estrada, Gabriel S. (2016) 'Ojibwe Lesbian Visual AIDS: On the Red Road with Carole laFavor, *Her Giveaway* (1988), and Native LGBTQ2 Film History,' *Journal of Lesbian Studies*, 20(3–4), 388–407.

Gilley, Brian J. (2014) 'Joyous Discipline: Native Autonomy and Culturally Conservative Two-Spirit People,' *American Indian Culture and Research Journal*, 38(2), 17–39. https://doi.org/10.17953/aicr.38.2.l874w4216151vp23

Grant, Jaime M., Motlett, Lisa and Tanis, Justin. (2011) *Injustice at Every Turn: A Report of the National Transgender Discrimination Survey*. Washington: National Center for Transgender Equality and National Gay and Lesbian Task Force. Available at: http://www.thetaskforce.org/injustice-every-turn-report-national-transgender-discrimination-survey/ [accessed on 26 February 2019].

Gross, Lawrence. (2014) *Anishinaabe Ways of Knowing and Being*. Farnham, UK: Ashgate Publishing.

Guerresio, Jason. (2012) 'Nanobah Becker, *Conversion*,' *Filmmaker: The Magazine of Independent Film*. Available at: http://filmmakermagazine.com/4889-nanobah-becker-writerdirector-conversion/ [accessed on 26 February 2019].

Knabe, Susan and Pearson, Wendy. (2013) 'Bash Back Baby, Your Life Depends on It: Pedagogical Responses to Anti-Gay Violence in John Greyson's *The Making of "Monsters"*,' in Longfellow, Brenda, MacKenzie, Scott and Waugh, Thomas (eds.), *The Perils of Pedagogy: The Works of John Greyson*. Montreal: McGill-Queen University Press, pp. 383–407.

Lewis, Randolph. (2012) *Navajo Talking Picture: Cinema on Native Ground*. Lincoln: University of Nebraska Press. https://doi.org/10.2307/j.ctt1d9nqn1

Marubbio, M. Elise. (2006) *Killing the Indian Maiden: Images of Native American Women in Film*. Lexington: The University Press of Kentucky. https://doi.org/10.5810/kentucky/9780813124148.001.0001

Million, Dian. (2013) *Therapeutic Nations: Healing in an Age of Indigenous Rights*. Tucson: University of Arizona Press.

Parker, Myra, Duran, Bonnie and Walters, Karina. (2017) 'The Relationship Between Bias-Related Victimization and Generalized Anxiety Disorder Among American Indian and Alaska Native Lesbian, Gay, Bisexual, Transgender, Two-Spirit Community Members,' *International Journal of Indigenous Health*, 12(2), 64–83. https://doi.org/10.18357/ijih122201717785

Pecore, Bradley. (2016) 'Bringing the Indigenous Queer Experience to Life in Fire Song,' *Logo NewNowNext*. Available at: http://www.newnownext.com/fire-song-native-adam-garnet-jones/11/2016/ [accessed on 26 February 2019].

Pitawanakwat, Lillian. (2006) 'Ojibwe Teaching.' Toronto: 4D Interactive Inc./ Invert Media and National Indigenous Literacy Association. Available at: www.fourdirectionsteachings.com [accessed on 26 February 2019].

Raheja, Michelle H. (2011) 'Visual Prophesies: *Imprint* and *It Starts with a Whisper*,' in Cummings, Denise K. (ed.), *Visualities: Perspectives on Contemporary American Indian Film and Art*. East Lansing: Michigan State University Press, pp. 3–40.

Sanchez, Casey. (2016) 'Love Among the Ruins: "Fire Song",' *Native Cinemas Showcase*. Available at: http://www.santafenewmexican.com/pasatiempo/movies/movie_reviews/love-among-the-ruins-fire-song/article_4958ed18-607a-5c77-a623-f331b4332b9c.html [accessed on 26 February 2019].

Shepardson, Mary. (1978) 'Changes in Navajo Mortuary Practices and Beliefs,' *American Indian Quarterly*, 4(4), 383–395. https://doi.org/10.2307/1184564

Waugh, Thomas. (2006) *The Romance of Transgression in Canada: Queering Sexualities, Nations, Cinemas*. Montreal: McGill-Queen's University Press.

Werito, Vincent. (2014) 'Understanding Hózhó to Achieve Critical Consciousness: A Contemporary Diné Interpretation of the Philosophical Principles of Hózhó,' in Lee, Lloyd L. (ed.), *Diné Perspectives Revitalizing and Reclaiming Navajo Thought*. Tucson: University of Arizona Press, pp. 25–38.

Zolbrod, Paul. (1987) *Diné Bahane': The Navajo Creation Story*. Albuquerque: University of New Mexico Press.

Tenured in American Indian Studies and promoted to Professor of Religious Studies at California State University (CSU) Long Beach, Gabriel S. Estrada holds a PhD in Comparative Cultural and Literary Studies from the University of Arizona at Tucson. Queer Indigenous media, Nahuatl language, and Indigenous literature are Dr Estrada's main areas of study. Co-Chair of the American Academy of Religion Indigenous Religious Traditions Unit, Dr Estrada is the author of 'Navajo Sci-Fi Film: Matriarchal Visual Sovereignty in Nanobah Becker's *The 6th World*' (*Journal of the American Academy of Religion*), 'Cloud Atlas' Queer Tiki Kitsch: Polynesia, Settler Colonialism, and Sci-Fi Film' (*Journal of Religion and Film*), 'Trans*lating the X in Caxcan and Xicanx Literature' in *Decolonizing Latinx Masculinities*, and is currently working on a book manuscript, *Two-Spirit Film Nepanta: Mediating Seven Trans*Indigenous Directions*. A two-spirit HIV+ scholar/activist and a Caxcan, Raramuri, Chiricahua Apache and Chicana/o descendant, Dr Estrada is Secretary of both Indigenous Pride LA and the City of Angeles Two-Spirit Society (CATSS).

Section Two

ALTERED STATES

Chapter 4

Sensing Reelism: Portals to Multiple Realities and Relationships in World, Indigenous and Documentary Cinema

LOUISE CHILD

At first glance, documentary cinema may appear to be the perfect medium for the teaching and research of lived religions. Rather than trying to imagine social and material worlds that can differ significantly from those of the student, documentary film seems to transport the viewer directly into those worlds to see religious practice in action. Most documentary films also have sound and one can therefore hear the spoken words of participants. Even if those words need to be translated, seeing and hearing them spoken on film offers viewers opportunities to observe facial expressions, body language and intonation in ways harder to convey by means of writing alone. The action of documentary films is immediate and contemporary to the time of their making and can therefore give the impression of at least in part fulfilling the agenda of lived religions as defined by Harvey in *Food, Sex and Strangers* (2013), i.e. recording what religious people actually do rather than focusing on textual prescriptions of ideal thought and behaviour. These advantages, however, present only a partial picture, and I will argue that a deeper engagement with the literatures of religious studies and sensorial anthropology can illuminate many of the problems associated with taking documentary film at face value. Further to this, I utilise a deeper examination of the limits and possibilities of the visual senses in film, arguing that critical engagement with world and indigenous fictional cinemas offers key insights into the role of storytelling in the transmission of numerous religious life-worlds. Moreover, the camera cannot capture directly many things that are seen with the 'mind's eye,' such as dreams and visions and also sightings of spirits and ghosts. This chapter therefore explores visual techniques in fictional films in order to suggest ways in which indigenous cinematic storytelling offers portals through which visions of spirits can be depicted.

THE LIMITATIONS OF VISUAL ANTHROPOLOGY

The medium of film is one primarily associated with the sense of sight. Senses of touch, taste and smell are not directly imprinted on and reproduced by celluloid, and although there have been important studies of sound in cinema (for example, Silverman 1988) these have arguably been less prominent than studies that examine frames, shots and picture compositions, partly perhaps because silent pictures preceded film, but also because of the ways in which sight has been given primacy in many scholastic and popular cultures that consider film. For example, visual anthropology appears to transport the viewer directly into the social world being examined; nonetheless, it is a constructed product that enables only limited sensual engagements. We hear and see films but we do not directly touch, taste or smell them. Moreover, the sensory engagements of anthropologists in the field are often continuous, spontaneous and unpredictable. Ethnographers are looked upon, smelt and touched: experiences that cannot be replicated by film but only alluded to.

Although the limitations of both observational realism in anthropology and neo-realism in the fictional cinema of Italy in the 1940s are well known (Grimshaw 2001: 71–89; Bondanella 2009 [2013]: 61–97; Haaland 2014) the tendency to assume that film can capture social reality persists. Scholars such as Carp (2008) have suggested that recent trends in scholarship of the senses are important for both explaining this phenomenon and providing a more balanced engagement with indigenous cultures for students and other audiences. He suggests that film's immediacy and immersion are potentially exciting and useful for students, but these qualities can also create the false impression that film transmits a form of unbiased truth, rather than reflecting the perceptions of scholars and editors. Carp (2008: 177) argues that 'as seductive as these materials are, they obfuscate religion and the religious even as they present them with impressive realism.' Therefore, in order for ethnographic film to 'offer students an opening onto a sophisticated consideration of religion and to the limitations and potentials of the means by which we study it,' two contexts should be introduced: sensorial anthropology and film theory as it relates to the anthropology of perception because 'it has become increasingly evident that perception varies significantly from culture to culture and within an individual culture' (Carp 2008: 178). Drawing from Classen (1998 and 1993), Carp argues that modern Western cultures' focus on the eye, using visuality as the primary source for metaphors, is a phenomenon that is linked to a reliance on text (Carp 2008: 179–180). He therefore suggests that, 'paradoxically, showing students films to break the hegemony of the text in some ways simply reinforces it' (2008: 181) and that it is important to help students break through this hegemony by engaging in meaningful ways with the idea that consciousness, self, senses and emotions are neither purely natural nor individual phenomena but are shaped by culture. Carp (2008: 181) uses as an example the fact that his students initially like and can easily accept Damascio's (1999: 11; 1994) explanation of consciousness as a 'movie in the brain.' He disrupts this comfort zone by asking them to read Guerts' (2005: 177) critique of this metaphor as anthropologically naive and bound by technological individualism; on doing so, students are flabbergasted to learn that the Anlo-Ewe of West Africa articulate consciousness as *sesalelame*, a kind of feeling in the body that is inherently intersubjective and rooted in shared feelings' (Carp 2008: 181). Carp therefore suggests that, 'once students grasp that others experience consciousness in quite a different way, they are ready to examine their own metaphors of consciousness. They quickly realize that "movie in the brain" as a metaphor for awareness could make sense only in a highly technologized and mediated culture' (Carp 2008: 181). He argues that it is important to engage students with the idea that making film is doing theory, and refers to Stoller's (1997; 1989) sensuous anthropological scholarship to suggest that 'it is not that people have sensory experience on the one side and understandings of it on another; rather, understandings (theology, ethics, spirituality and so forth) are part and parcel of sensory experience' (Carp 2008: 184, 185), an insight that is also critical to Harvey's (2013) challenges to the 'religion as belief' model.

Rather than conceiving of film as a 'window to the world,' therefore, I suggest that when film is examined in the light of sensorial anthropology, radical transformations in understandings of personhood become possible, akin to Meyer and Land's (2003) threshold concepts. Drawing inspiration from Turner's (1969) work on liminality, Meyer and Land (2003: 1) examine the ways in which students may find particular forms of disciplinary knowledge difficult if it runs counter to previous ways of doing things or apprehending the world. They suggest the term 'threshold concept' for this kind of knowledge and argue that it is like 'a portal, opening up a new and previously inaccessible way of thinking about something.' While Meyer and Land's theories have been applied to a wide range of disciplinary learning, they are particularly provocative when considering perspectives and worldviews of diverse cultures (Abbott and Child 2015). The work of Lutz (1988), for example, makes a close study of emotion words and their usage by the people of a small South Pacific island called Ifaluk in order to suggest very different conceptions of anger on the island to those typical of America and Western Europe. She argues that emotions are neither purely natural nor individual phenomena. Moreover, different cultures do not just have different words for the same emotions, but emotional responses are themselves constituted through the social dynamics of societies and the ways in which their members are socialised through emotion terms (Lutz 1988: 81). Exploring these ideas with students therefore leads to some fundamental and interesting questions that can destabilise assumptions about their own social worlds and fundamental ideas about personhood, and therefore are good examples of 'portalling' phenomena.

In another example, Capps' (1976) *Seeing with a Native Eye* and Morrison (1992) argue that understanding the world from a Native American perspective involves fundamental reorientations of perception, many of which stem from the ways in which their religions govern relationships between human beings and with animals, the environment and spirits. Gross (2016 [2012]: 80–120) develops this idea with a careful analysis of Anishinaabe language, arguing that engaging with this language is not simply a matter of translating terms into English (and by extension a cause-and-effect model of understanding time and action) but rather taking on a quantum worldview in which process and relationship are key.

As Hume (2007: 2–3) suggests, 'the "sensuous awakening" (Stoller 1997: xii) that has occurred within certain sectors of anthropology is providing us with more juicy, vibrant, sensual and exciting ethnographic accounts that take us into the field to experience the smells and feelings of what it is to actually "be there" or to imagine other historical epochs in all their tasteful and distasteful glory.' Hume uses the concept of portals to explore ways in which ritual practices may stimulate the senses and thereby provide a gateway to altered states of consciousness. Exploring this 'cross-culturally common mystical experience called portalling— moving from one reality to another via a tunnel, door, aperture, hole or the like' (Hume 2007: 6), she points to various techniques of portal creation, including song, dance and the creation of specialised diagrams, such as mandalas and yantras. It is significant that all of these techniques have sensual dimensions and that, furthermore, the transformations of consciousness associated with them are often radical and profound. She suggests that 'the everyday reality that we perceive through our senses can be altered dramatically by "working" the senses using a variety of somatic stimuli, creating a paradigm shift in perception' that is akin to going through a portal (Hume 2007: 1).

This idea is depicted in the film *Dreamkeeper* (2003), which uses live action and special effects to recount a number of stories in which spirits (including, for example, coyote and spider trickster spirits) are important characters. One tale, *Legend of Eagle Boy's Vision Quest*, opens the film, and it centres on a young man seeking a vision quest by going without food and water for four days. In a scene where the boy confronts (unwisely we learn later) the mountain spirits, the mountainside becomes increasingly animated: steam appears as if from a geyser, rocks chase him down the mountainside and he is sucked into a hole. Eyes appear in the mountain, which appears to morph into the shape of a wolf. In another tale, the spirit Thunderbird falls in love with a woman and transports her into his world. In his realm, he appears as a handsome man, but in her earthly world he manifests as storms. In this film the process of storytelling itself acts like a portal, and its sacred nature is signified by the fact that when the grandfather is telling a story he picks up his drum.

THE TRUTHS OF FICTION

Storytelling (whether of myths or personal histories) often plays an important part in teaching for indigenous peoples. In one example, Guédon (2012 [1994]) explores storytelling as a method of transmitting 'Dene Ways,' a term that covers a range of cultural knowledge among the Dene of inland Alaska and northwestern Canada. She explains that although the stories were broadly stable entities, in practice their telling was responsive to and tailored towards individuals' questions, situations that arose, and the level of understanding that the listeners were deemed to have (Guédon 2012 [1994]: 44). This raises two points in relation to the potential for indigenous film to tell stories (and thereby transmit religious and cultural knowledge) effectively. On the one hand, it suggests that for many indigenous peoples to communicate about their own cultures, visual storytelling, as well as documentary, would be important. However, film is disadvantaged compared to storytelling in an interpersonal context because there are less subtle and fluid interactions between the story and its audiences. Some indigenous films such as *Dreamkeeper* (2003) compensate for this issue by depicting the process of storytelling itself and demonstrating examples of how choices of stories are influenced by social and personal context. In *Dreamkeeper*, a seventeen-year-old Lakota man called Shane Chasing Horse reluctantly accompanies his grandfather, Pete Chasing Horse, from the Pine Ridge Reservation where they live to his last All Nations Pow Wow. Along the way, Pete Chasing Horse tells a number of stories that are relevant to incidents in their journey and recounts in instalments the Lakota *Legend of Eagle Boy's Vision Quest*, which is the story that mirrors Shane's (Harper 2010).

The physical situation in which indigenous storytelling takes place is also important. Guédon (2012 [1994]: 45–46) suggests that an acquisition of intimate knowledge of the land 'is the inclusion of the land itself into the cultural environment and process. This factor was paramount in my own socialization process, as well as that of Nabesna children. It is in the bush...that I was taught most of the techniques, stories, rituals, and traditions concerning animals and the environment at large, the earth and the winds, the mountains and the rivers and the proper attitude toward them': a statement that echoes the concern with everyday activities and interspecies relationships in Harvey's (2013: 2) definition of religion. Guédon goes on to explain how the richness of meaning is continually embedded within the environment through the stories of what happens to individual community members in particular places. Engagement with place can also highlight specific features of indigenous filmmaking and the limitations of this visual medium. Some indigenous films include extensive long shots of the environment so that, in one sense, the land itself can be regarded as a character. Nonetheless, the fixed nature of film means that each film is only one telling of a story. It can be evocative, but cannot replicate the multisensory, ever developing experience of a day-to-day engagement with land and community that Guédon describes.

Third, Guédon discusses the importance of dreaming in the shamanic activity of the Dene, a people who do recognise expert practitioners but who also acknowledge the significance of dreaming for members of the wider community. She explains that her own dreams became more vivid and clear during her fieldwork period and that her discussion of her dreams was an important part of the process by which she was offered more knowledge and responsibility within the group. Noting the differences between her previous understandings of dreams as representations or symbols and the ways in which they were understood by the Dene, Guédon points to the ways in which the normal cultural boundaries between humans and animals can be dissolved in dreams and also to the attention paid by the Dene to how dreams feel, 'as an anticipation of a real experience...perceived by the body' (2012 [1994]: 57–58). Although film as a visual medium is limited in its capacity to convey these bodily sensations and emotional states in dreams, there are, nonetheless, interesting examples of indigenous filmmakers who explore dreaming, mythology and landscapes from indigenous points of view. In so doing, their films can act to some extent as portals not only to altered states of consciousness, but also provide lenses through which different ways of seeing the world can be portrayed.

DREAMS, MYTHS AND STORYTELLING

One of the challenges facing indigenous filmmakers in their transmission of myths or dreams onto fictional films is the fact that, although both myths and dreams may be associated with sight, many cultures regard storytelling as an activity that is spoken and heard, while some societies, such as the Andamanese, may examine smells in dreams in considerable detail (Vishvajit 2004). Nonetheless, Kracke (1992: 31–32) argues that both myth and dream telling contain the construction of vivid images that depend 'on inner visualisation for [their] communication and impact; thus, myths are constituted in a spatial-sensory modality like that of dreams.'

In one example, the film *Atanarjuat*, by an Inuit director, Zacharias Kunuk, received considerable critical acclaim for its innovative visual style. As Wood (2008: 144) suggests, 'the on-screen look of *Atanarjuat: The Fast Runner* was self-consciously crafted to present a visual equivalent of the oral tale upon which it is based.' The choice to film this particular bedtime story sprang from Kunuk's recognition that the tale contained, at heart, an especially arresting visual image. As Kunuk explains: 'Once you get that picture into your head of that naked man running for his life across the sea ice, his hair flying, you never forget it. It had everything for a fantastic movie—love, jealousy, murder and revenge, and at the same time, buried in this ancient Inuit "action thriller" were all these lessons we kids were supposed to learn about how if you break these taboos that kept our ancestors alive, you could be out there running for your life, just like him' (Kunuk, quoted in White 2005: 62 and re-quoted in Wood 2008: 134). Wood goes on to suggest that although the murder and the chase that follow it form the film's narrative core, this core 'is more deeply rooted in a pre-modern Inuit epic than in commercial cinema. The chase abruptly and surprisingly transforms the pace of the film, which until that moment likely seems to most non-Inuit audiences to be moving forward very slowly, more like an ethnography or a documentary than a feature film. The violence and terror surrounding the chase sequence abruptly infuse new meanings into the long, meditative scenes that have come before. In addition, Atanarjuat's run concludes in a fundamentally Inuit manner, through guidance from a spirit and then a magical leap over a wide crack in the ice' (Wood 2008: 135).

This later point raises the issue of how one might depict spirit beings in indigenous film. Evans (2010: 19–31) examines this question in some detail, pointing to the interest in ethnographic authenticity of Kunuk and other producers of the film and the ways this includes spiritual authenticity and depictions of 'unseen realms' (p. 19). This concern is partly because the story arc of the original legend takes place in both human and spirit spheres. The first scene in which this becomes evident involves an evil shaman, Tuurngarjuaq, who has been invited by one of the camp's members because the latter wishes to displace its current leader. A spiritual battle between the camp's leader, Kumaglak, and the shaman is depicted by showing both men tied with ropes (to restrict their physical powers and throw the battle into the spiritual realm) and focusing on their contorted expressions and grunting sounds which indicate the conflict between their walrus and polar bear spirit helpers (Evans 2010: 20). In another scene which shows an attack on Atanarjuat and his brother years later, a ghostly voice interrupts the attackers and they see the ghost of Kumaglak, a frightening event that buys Atanarjuat just enough time to make his escape running naked on the ice (Evans 2010: 20–21).

In the case of *Atanarjuat*, therefore, the choice is for a style of live action narrative set in a pre-colonial era that, Raheja argues, both draws from and subverts conventions of ethnographies such as *Nanook of the North*. While *Atanarjuat* similarly draws attention to the spectacular landscapes of the Inuit, and their day-to-day engagement with these to survive, the Inuit characters, far from being the 'happy go lucky' men and women depicted in Flaherty's *Nanook*, are morally ambiguous and complex (Raheja 2010: 209). The film also combines themes and techniques that have proved appealing to multiple audiences (European, Native and non-Native American) with a style that requires more work from non-Inuit audiences. Although the story is a myth, the characters speak in their native language (with European subtitles), there is no voiceover and the identity of shamanic or spirit characters is not obvious to audience members unfamiliar with the story, who must therefore turn to supplementary books and other materials put together by the filmmaking team to learn more (Raheja 2010: 210–213; Angilirq, Kunuk, Paniaq and Qulitalik 2002).

Another consequence of this kind of depiction is to suggest that shamans and spirits are not necessarily easily distinguished by appearance. There are, however, examples which make this point but also depict the context in which stories are told. Unlike with face-to-face encounters, films remain the same each time and place they are shown. However, some indigenous films show an interaction between stories and those who tell and hear them by using the device of stories within stories. In one short example, *Maq and the Spirit of the Woods* (2006), directed by Phyllis Grant, the story itself is animated but there are short sequences that introduce and close the film using live actors. It opens with a Native man (played by Gilbert Sewell) telling a story to a group of children in the woods. He is carrying a drum (which suggests that playing this instrument is going to be part of the storytelling process). The story is about a Mi'kmaq boy who is often clumsy. An elder offers him a small piece of pipe stone, explaining that this stone is special and that when a pipe is made out of it, the smoke from that pipe carries the prayers of the smoker to the creator. Maq decides to make a person out of the stone, and pleased with his efforts, he sets off on a path through the woods to show it to his grandfather who lives on the other side. As he journeys through the woods he meets another traveller named Mi'gmwesu, spending three happy days and nights with him eating and swapping stories. During this time the little stone figure glows. Once the boy reaches his grandfather the latter explains that the boy had set off only two hours ago and that Mi'gmwesu is actually the spirit of the woods. He advises the boy to keep the stone with him at all times. At the end of the film we return to the live person group with which the film began and the man shows the stone to the children. Thus the film suggests important connections between the world of the story and the world in which stories are told and received. At the same time, it suggests that spirit beings may look just like human persons but that engagement with spirits and the places they inhabit (such as the woods) may take place in altered realities and time frames.

In another example, this time from New Zealand, *Kaitangata Twitch* (based on a book by Mahy [2005]), the whole story is set in the present although events and characters from both the mythical world and the historical past enter the story with agency and engage in interesting ways with its central protagonist, twelve-year-old Meredith Gallagher. Meredith lives with her family—father Carey, mother Grace, older sister Kate and younger brother Rufus—in a small rural town next to a mysterious island called Kaitangata. Both the family and the town as a whole have complex relationships with the island and with environmental issues more broadly, issues that crystallise in the story around the development plans of a business-man called Sebastian Cardwell. The television series avoids simple divisions along racial lines as Meredith's parents are depicted as having both European (Carey) and Maori (Grace) heritage and Grace's ancestors are said to belong to the tribe that has the longest and closest history of engagement with the local area. Sebastian Cardwell, however, is also Maori, and is able to speak Maori language. Nonetheless, the primary storyline and a number of filmic techniques indicate this programme is deeply influenced by Maori spirituality in the sense that Hardy (2012: 11) suggests as films 'which are also shaped by indigenous behaviour in relation to the spiritual energies diffused through human life and the natural world' (see also Child 2015; Hardy 2003).

This spiritual orientation is most evident through Meredith's relationship with the island, which is expressed, for example, through strange dreams; the island responding to her playing a flute, and her seeing scenes and people from the past there. This relationship is at first discouraged by an old Maori, Lee Kaa, who expresses anger and concern that Meredith and her playmates do not obey proper protocols because they do not understand that the island is both sacred and dangerous. However, as the series progresses Lee becomes a mentor for Meredith, warning her that he knows Kaitangata is speaking to her and that her dreams are powerful but not safe, because it is not simply that she dreams about the island but that the island uses dreams to bond with her. He explains, 'the dream is an in between place. Don't let it catch you in its dreams. You'll be caught between two worlds.' This is because the island is also the spirit of a cannibal chief who experiences hunger and anger when disturbed. This is depicted in one scene where builders are drilling into a rock on the island. The ground starts shaking and Meredith falls and hits her head, bleeding while the ground beneath her opens to reveal a mouth-like aperture that swallows her blood. In addition to animating the myth of the cannibal chief, the programme also shows Meredith engaging with spirits from the historical past. She sees the spirit of a girl, Shelly Gentry, who disappeared fifty years ago and who tries to help Meredith build a harmonious relationship with the island. Meredith also sees the spirits of Maori people from the more distant past in front of an animated cave that tries to swallow them. At several points in the story the image of the face of the cannibal chief is superimposed subtly onto the image of the cave to signify that they are one and the same person. The island is therefore a place that acts like a portal both for ancestral and mythical beings and for ghosts, but the story remains firmly in the present while engaging in exciting ways with both the past and the spiritual dimensions of the landscape. This combination creates an interesting tension because while negotiation with ancestral and land spirits often entails practices aimed at continually taking care of a relationship with these beings to maintain harmony, the entrance of a ghost is often suggestive in narrative of an intrusion into the present of an aspect of the past that cannot ever be truly resolved.

TEMPORAL PORTALS: GHOSTS, TRAUMA AND ETHICAL COMMUNITIES

In exploring both deities connected to the land and ghosts with very personal connections to the living, *Kaitangata Twitch* combines in very subtle and interesting ways complex connections to the colonial past in New Zealand and visions of a future that embraces environmental issues and Maori traditions in dynamic and diverse ways. While many of the spirits that I have explored in this chapter are of a more collective, religious character, in that they embody environmental and other deities, ghosts in American films (especially comedy romances) are often spirits of the dead who return to resolve very personal issues with particular loved ones (Child forthcoming 2020). Nonetheless, there has been an increasing development of academic interest in depictions of ghosts and their significance for cultural theory and collective memory (Gordon 2008; Del Pilar Blanco and Peeren 2013). Particularly when these investigations are related to the study of collective trauma (Kaplan 2005), they can shed light on how ghosts on film illuminate collective emotions about the traumatic echoes of past repressive political regimes.

Compelling examples of this kind of study can be found in examinations of Spanish films made subsequent to the regime of Franco, such as Gutiérrez-Albilla's work on trauma in the cinema of the Spanish director Pedro Almodóvar, a director whose work famously spans the end of the Franco dictatorship in Spain and celebrates complex and rapid social changes that followed it, particularly in Madrid in the 1980s and 1990s. While there are many comic elements to Almodóvar's work, Gutiérrez-Albilla is particularly interested in the ways in which it expresses incomplete processes of mourning and working through collective traumas in that society. Although not advocating a depressive, melancholic position, Gutiérrez-Albilla (2017: 19–20) aims to 'foreground the impossibility of complete working through in order to articulate an affirmation of the ethical and political potential of mourning, both subjectively and politically.' In his analysis of *Volver*, a film in which the central character's mother both is, and is not, a ghost, Gutiérrez-Albilla foregrounds sensual cinematic strategies such as tensions between motion and stillness and evocation of smell to explain how film can conjure spectres who embody and play out complex and incomplete processes of collective grief. While neither Franco nor his regime are explicitly discussed in *Volver*, the traces of the impact of his rule are evoked through the characters of the father of the central female character, Raimunda, and her husband, both of whom are guilty of abusive crimes that can be linked to patriarchal authority.

For Gutiérrez-Albilla, (2017: 44) the absent-present ghosts in *Volver* are not only there to explore personal emotions, but also bring to our attention to the fact that 1980s democratic, modern Spain is 'a society predicated on the disavowal of the spectres of the traumatic past' and reveal in subtle ways 'the horrors to which national identity was subjected under Francoism.' Attempts to disavow or move past fascism without proper acknowledgement of the psychic wounds it inflicted on the nation may be convenient for modern nation-states, but the traces remain in dominant patriarchal ideologies of Spanish society. Moreover he suggests, drawing from Labanyi (2007), that fictional ghosts can reveal 'the spectral past's intoxicating effects in the present' more effectively than documentaries because the documentary can offer audiences the relief of distance while horror fiction and the ghost film are more slippery, subtle and evocative in their effects, offering spaces for audiences to work through collective traumas without enforcing premature closure or denial of the past (Gutiérrez-Albilla 2017: 45).

Moreover, ghosts do more than offer the living a more complete history; according to Lim (2001), they disrupt the paradigms of conventional linear histories and the power dynamics associated with them. Lim argues that 'the temporality of haunting, through which events and people return from the limits of time and mortality, differs sharply from the modern concept of a linear, progressive, universal time. The hauntings recounted by ghost narratives are not merely instances of the past reasserting itself in a stable present, as it is usually assumed; on the contrary, the ghostly return of traumatic events precisely troubles the boundaries of past, present, and future' (Lim 2001: 287). It is this potential for paradigm shifts that leads me to suggest that ghost narratives have qualities akin to the other portals explored in this chapter, where understanding persons and relationships in societies with different sensory and emotional paradigms to one's own entails radical shifts in orientation to knowledge and the world and ultimately transformations in oneself. Examples of ghost sightings and stories in societies impacted by colonialism are thereby doubly interesting, in that they can both provide insights into the long-term and continuing impacts of the colonial encounter itself. Gross (2016 [2012]: 33–51) characterises these impacts upon the Native American Anishinaabeg people as 'postapocalypse stress syndrome,' while at the same time highlighting indigenous conceptions of time and space that may differ, contrast and challenge linear, hegemonic assertions of 'the historical' by colonial powers. Scholars such as Landrum (2011: 271–272) explore the importance of returning Native American spiritual objects and remains of the dead 'held hostage' in museums to their tribes. While this is a question of respect and countering spiritual colonialism, these items are also considered to be charged with activity, manifesting ghostly sounds in the museums and adversely affecting the health of descendants unable to perform spiritual duties to the remains. In another example, she refers to ghostly apparitions at the site of the Wounded Knee Massacre of 1989 (Pine Ridge Reservation in South Dakota). She explains that, 'it is common knowledge among the Sioux that the dead walk at night, particularly at that location, because of the emotional trauma that was imprinted on the land. They also believe that the land is timeless and that lines between the past and the present, the day-to-day and the supernatural, are skewed, rather than neatly drawn' (Landrum 2011: 264).

Nonetheless, although ghost stories may be helpful for Native Americans coming to terms with the traumatic effects of colonialism, scholars such as Bergland (2013: 372–373) highlight the dangers of this strategy, because the 'myth of the vanishing Indian' implies a total conquest of Native American peoples, allowing the national consciousness to indulge in a cosy sense of guilt rather than engaging with modern Native American peoples who have not only survived but are building positive futures.

Raheja (2010: 145) concurs with this caution with regard to this trope, stating that 'the image of the ghostly Indian as a figment of an American imagination invested in Native Americans as spectral entities of a tragic and mostly elided past within a broader field of historical amnesia.... Native Americans become apparitional excesses in the dominant culture's repressed imagination, which seems perpetually unable to confront the violence of its founding.' She therefore suggests that we turn to the work of indigenous filmmakers for ghosts who do more than simply provide a place for fleeting guilt about historical colonial injustice that can thereby be quickly forgotten at the end of the film. Instead of relegating Native

Americans to a tragic past, modern indigenous filmmakers are challenging the trope of the ghostly Indian with creative play and attention to the embodied present of Native peoples (Raheja 2010: 146).

The film *Imprint*, produced by Cheyenne and Arapaho filmmaker Chris Eyre and directed by Michael Linn, is set on Pine Ridge Reservation in South Dakota, a site significant as the setting for the Wounded Knee Massacre and the cemetery where victims are buried. Raheja asserts, however, that the film both refers to the horrors at Wounded Knee and evokes a vibrant Lakota future rather than simply replicating the problems associated with the 'kind of nostalgic, past tense vision of Indigenous culture that bolsters the myth of the vanishing Indian' (Raheja 2010: 147). Rather than conforming to expectations of either ghost story or Western genres, *Imprint* has a strong female *Lakota* woman as the central protagonist and plays in exciting ways with ideas about ghosts, spirits, prophecy and time.

According to Raheja, spirituality and epistemic Indigenous knowledges are key ways in which *Imprint* challenges both images of the static ghostly Indian and Western understandings of time, history and prophecy. As an example of the creativity of what she calls 'the virtual reservation,' these challenges do not fall back on promises of accessing 'authentic' or mystical Native practices for the pleasures of non-Native audiences but demonstrate complex and multilayered engagements of modern indigenous peoples from a range of perspectives including gender (Raheja 2010: 49). Nonetheless, spirits and the spiritual are considered to be 'a vibrant and integral part of human existence' for a number of indigenous activists and scholars who link their importance with threats to Judeo-Christian understandings of gender, the primacy of written narrative and 'Western conceptions of temporality' (Raheja 2010: 158).

Imprint achieves this by defying audience expectations about the strange shadow shapes that Shayla, a Lakota lawyer, sees when she returns to her parents' ranch. The film explores ghostly possibilities, suggesting that the haunting may be by her brother who is missing (presumed dead), or the troubled spirits of Lakota people murdered during the Wounded Knee Massacre (Raheja 2010: 163–164). Her suspicions are further fuelled by her father, Sam, drawing an image of an individual hanged in a barn, which Shayla believes may be a confession of his son's murder. However, a medicine man called in to help casts doubt on this interpretation by telling her that 'past, present, and future all touch each other. Time doesn't exist. For spirits, time doesn't exist.' This turns out to be the key to resolving the mystery and to the twist that makes this a unique ghost movie.

Rather than looking only to the past, the film's climax suggests Shayla's predictive powers, as the shadows are actually of an attempted murder of her future self by a fellow attorney (Jonathan) who is worried that she might discover that he fabricated a recent case. The image her father drew is of Shayla saving herself in the barn by becoming entangled with a hook while Jonathan plunges to his death. Therefore, while Wounded Knee is not forgotten in the film, it is, nonetheless, Shayla's abilities to perceive more deeply, defend herself and forge a future that are its overarching themes.

While indigenous films may contribute to the working through of collective traumas, therefore, we should also be aware of the creative ways in which they participate in contemporary exploration and resistance (Rader 2011). While film's association with sight potentially makes this medium problematic because of the historic tendency to equate seeing with knowing in hegemonic and rationalistic ways, film can also be a medium for evocative and imaginative storytelling, and as such is well suited as a vehicle through which to explore and introduce indigenous spirit persons to traditional and broader audiences. This is partly because even so-called 'live action' films are in fact animated art forms. Animated films such as *Maq and the Spirit of the Woods* convey well the idea that engagements with spirits may take place in portals (such as the woods) within which there are alternative experiences of the passage of time. Similarly, the island in the *Kaitangata Twitch* is animated by a spirit and is itself a portal that can swallow human beings, both as flesh and more subtly through dream relationships in which the island has agency and can penetrate human individuals. Its portal capacity is also vitally temporal, giving access to persons from the historical past (fifty years ago), the ancestral past and mythical atemporal dimensions. Time, space and landscape are therefore not simply folded but radically reconceived through this type of narrative which can reflect and explore religious life-worlds that include spirit beings.

Rader (2011: 152–153) makes important observations in the Native American context about the ways in which her term 'virtual reservation' captures both the injustices of colonial history in America and the ways in which modern indigenous filmmakers are vibrantly present. Moreover, she suggests that this is a space that maintains 'a dialectical relationship between the multiple layers of Indigenous knowledge systems—from the dream world to the topography of real and imagined landscapes.' Indigenous films can therefore both honour and re-present traditional ways of seeing while at the same time embodying a contemporary art form that is open to change with the artistic skills and social and political experiences of each generation. As such they are a testament to the living religions in the present as well as a medium for capturing traditional and mythical pasts.

FILMOGRAPHY

Atanarjuat: The Fast Runner. (2001) Directed by Z. Kunuk.
Dreamkeeper. (2003) Directed by S. Barron.
Imprint. (2007) Directed by M. Linn.
Kaitangata Twitch. (2010) Directed by Y. McKay.
Maq and the Spirit of the Woods. (2006) Directed by P. Grant.
Nanook of the North. (1922) Directed by R. Flaherty.
Volver. (2006) Directed by P. Almodóvar.

REFERENCES

Abbott, S. and Child, L. (2015) 'Learning via the Liminal: Portals, Transformation and Indigenous Arts' (conference paper), *Re-enchanting the Academy*. Canterbury: Christchurch University, UK, 25–27 September.

Angiliriq, P. A., Kunuk, Z., Paniaq, H. and Qulitalik, P. (eds.) (2002) *Atanarjuat: The Fast Runner*. Toronto: Coach House & Isuma.

Bergland, R. L. (2013) 'Indian Ghosts and American Subjects' (extract from *The National Uncanny: Indian Ghosts and American Subjects*, University Press of New England), in Del Pilar Blanco, M. and Peeren, E. (eds.), *The Spectralities Reader: Ghosts and Haunting in Contemporary Cultural Theory*. London: Bloomsbury, pp. 371–392.

Bondanella, P. (2013 [2009]) *A History of Italian Cinema*. London: Bloomsbury. https://doi.org/10.1093/obo/9780199791286-0107

Capps, W. H. (ed.) (1976) *Seeing with a Native Eye: Essays on Native American Religion*. New York: Harper & Row.

Carp, R. (2008) 'Seeing Is Believing, but Touching's the Truth: Religion, Film, and the Anthropology of the Senses,' in Watkins, G. J. (ed.), *Teaching Religion and Film*. Oxford: Oxford University Press.
https://doi.org/10.1093/acprof:oso/9780195335989.003.0014

Child, L. (2015) 'Maori Arts as Film Art: An Analysis of Ritual and Myth in *Whale Rider*, *Once Were Warriors* and *Te Rua*,' *DISKUS (The Journal of the British Association for the Study of Religion)*, 17(3), 1–17.

Child, L. (forthcoming 2020) *Dreams, Vampires and Ghosts: Anthropological Perspectives on the Sacred and Psychology in Film and Television*. London: Bloomsbury.

Classen, C. (1993) *Worlds of Sense: Exploring the Senses in History and across Cultures*. New York: Routledge.

Classen, C. (1998) *The Color of Angels: Cosmology, Gender, and the Aesthetic Imagination*. New York: Routledge.

Damascio, A. R. (1994) *Descartes' Error: Emotion, Reason and the Human Brain*. New York: Avon Books Inc.

Damascio, A. R. (1999) *The Feeling of What Happens: Body and Emotion in the Making of Consciousness*. San Diego and New York: Harcourt Inc.

Del Pilar Blanco, M. and Peeren, E. (eds.) (2013) *The Spectralities Reader: Ghosts and Haunting in Contemporary Cultural Theory*. London: Bloomsbury.

Evans, M. R. (2010) *The Fast Runner: Filming the Legend of Atanarjuat*. Lincoln, NB: University of Nebraska Press. https://doi.org/10.2307/j.ctt1dfnrh3

Gordon, A. F. (2008) *Ghostly Matters: Haunting and the Sociological Imagination*. Minneapolis: University of Minnesota Press.

Grimshaw, A. (2001) *The Ethnographer's Eye: Ways of Seeing in Anthropology*. Cambridge: Cambridge University Press. https://doi.org/10.1017/CBO9780511817670

Gross, L.W. (2016 [2012]) *Anishaabe Ways of Knowing and Being*. Abingdon, UK: Routledge.

Guédon, M. F. (2012 [1994]) 'Dene Ways and the Ethnographer's Culture,' in Young, D. E. and J. (eds.) *Being Changed by Cross-Cultural Encounters: The Anthropology of Extraordinary Experience*. Toronto: University of Toronto Press, pp. 39–70. https://doi.org/10.3138/9781442602366-003

Guerts, K. L. (2005) 'Consciousness as "Feeling in the Body": A West African Theory of Embodiment, Emotion and the Making of Mind,' in Howes, D. (ed.), *Empire of the Senses: The Sensual Culture Reader*. London: Bloomsbury, pp. 164–178.

Gutiérrez-Albilla, J. D. (2017) *Aesthetics, Ethics and Trauma in the Cinema of Pedro Almodóvar*. Edinburgh: Edinburgh University Press.

Haaland, T. (2014) *Italian Neorealist Cinema*. Edinburgh: Edinburgh University Press.

Hardy, A. (2003) 'Return of the Taniwha: The Re-Spiritualization of Land and Film in Aotearoa,' *British Review of New Zealand Studies*, 14, 87–104.

Hardy, A. (2012) 'Hidden Gods – Religion, Spirituality and Recent New Zealand Cinema,' *Studies in Australasian Cinema*, 6(1), 11–27. https://doi.org/10.1386/sac.6.1.11_1

Harper, F. (2010) 'Walking the Good Red Road: Storytelling in the Counselling Relationship Using the Film *Dreamkeeper*,' *Journal of Creativity in Mental Health*, 5(2), 216–220. https://doi.org/10.1080/15401383.2010.485119

Harvey, G. (2013) *Food, Sex, and Strangers: Understanding Religion as Everyday Life*. Durham: Acumen. https://doi.org/10.4324/9781315729572

Howes, D. (ed.) (2005) *Empire of the Senses: The Sensual Culture Reader*. London: Bloomsbury.

Hume, L. (2007) *Portals: Opening Doorways to Other Realities through the Senses*. Oxford: Berg.

Kaplan, E. A. (2005) *Trauma Culture: The Politics of Terror and Loss in Media and Literature*. New Brunswick, NJ: Rutgers University Press.

Kracke, W. (1992) 'Myth in Dreams, Thought in Images: An Amazonian Contribution to the Psychoanalytic Theory of Primary Process,' in Tedlock, B. (ed.), *Dreaming: Anthropological and Psychological Interpretations*. Santa Fe, NM: School of American Research Press, pp. 31–54.

Labanyi, J. (2007) 'Memory and Modernity in Democratic Spain: The Difficulty of Coming to Terms with the Spanish Civil War,' *Poetics Today*, 28(1), 89–116. https://doi.org/10.1215/03335372-2006-016

Landrum, C. (2011) 'Shape-shifters, Ghosts, and Residual Power: An Examination of Northern Plains Spiritual Beliefs, Location, Objects, and Spiritual Colonialism,' in Boyd, C. E. and Thrush, C. (eds.), *Phantom Past, Indigenous Presence: Native Ghosts in North American Culture and History*. Lincoln: University of Nebraska Press, pp. 255–279. https://doi.org/10.2307/j.ctt1df4h07.14

Lim, B. C. (2001) 'Spectral Times: The Ghost Film as Historical Allegory,' *Positions*, 9(2), 287–329. https://doi.org/10.1215/10679847-9-2-287

Lutz, C. (1988) *Unnatural Emotions: Everyday Sentiments on a Micronesian Atoll and Their Challenge to Western Theory*. Chicago: The University of Chicago Press. https://doi.org/10.7208/chicago/9780226219783.001.0001

Mahy, M. (2005) *Kaitangata Twitch*. Crow's Nest, NSW: Allen & Unwin.

Meyer, J. and Land, R. (2003) 'Threshold Concepts and Troublesome Knowledge: Linkages to Ways of Thinking and Practising within the Disciplines,' *Enhanced Teaching-Learning Environments in Undergraduate Courses, Occasional Report 4*. Edinburgh: University of Edinburgh.

Morrison, K. M. (1992) 'Beyond the Supernatural: Language and Religious Action,' *Religion*, 2, 201–205. https://doi.org/10.1016/0048-721X(92)90016-W

Rader, D. (2011) *Engaged Resistance: American Indian Art, Literature, and Film from Alcatraz to the NMAI*. Austin: University of Texas Press.

Raheja, M. H. (2010) *Reservation Reelism: Redfacing, Visual Sovereignty and Representations of Native Americans in Film*. Lincoln, NB: University of Nebraska Press. https://doi.org/10.2307/j.ctt1dfnrq6

Silverman, K. (1988) *The Acoustic Mirror: The Female Voice in Psychoanalysis and Cinema*. Bloomington and Indianapolis: Indiana University Press.

Stoller, P. (1989) *The Taste of Ethnographic Things: The Senses in Anthropology*. Philadelphia: University of Pennsylvania Press. https://doi.org/10.9783/9780812203141

Stoller, P. (1997) *Sensuous Scholarship*. Philadelphia: University of Pennsylvania Press. https://doi.org/10.9783/9780812203134

Turner, V. (1969) *The Ritual Process: Structure and Anti-Structure*. New York: Aldine De Gruyter.

Vishvajit, P. (2004) 'Forest Smells and Spider Webs: Ritualized Dream Interpretation among Andaman Islanders,' *Dreaming*, 14, 136–150. https://doi.org/10.1037/1053-0797.14.2-3.136

White, J. (2005) 'Frozen but Always in Motion: Arctic Film, Video, and Broadcast,' *Velvet Light Trap*, 55, 52–64. https://doi.org/10.1353/vlt.2005.0010

Wood, H. (2008) *Native Features: Indigenous Films from around the World*. London: Bloomsbury. https://doi.org/10.5040/9781628928815

Dr Louise Child is a lecturer in myth, ritual and film studies at Cardiff University, UK, with research interests in altered states of consciousness including dreams, visions, mysticism, shamanism and possession trance, and their depictions in popular and indigenous films. She is a member of the British Association for the Study of Religion and has published on indigenous film in New Zealand for their journal. Her book *Tantric Buddhism and Altered States of Consciousness: Durkheim, Emotional Energy and Visions of the Consort* has recently been reissued in paperback by Routledge. She is currently working on a second book project, *Dreams, Vampires and Ghosts: Anthropological Perspectives on the Sacred and Psychology in Film and Television*.

Chapter 5

The Female Gaze: Sight and the Medusa Myth

GINA BEVAN

Sight is a central theme within the ancient myth of Medusa, whose petrifying gaze could turn those who looked at her to stone. For this reason, the Gorgon was a popular apotropaic icon and her image was ubiquitous in the ancient Greek world. She is often found on the antefix of temples dedicated to various Olympian deities as a protector of those sacred spaces. Medusa is usually depicted on these temples with her head turned directly to meet the gaze of passers-by with her bulbous eyes, and thus art historian Mark Stansbury-O'Donnell likens her to cult statues of deities that were designed to look out at the mortal viewer as an 'epiphany, a visualization of the divine that engages the viewer' (2015: 185). Whereas looking at *statues* of the Gorgon and the gods was 'safe,' gazing upon Medusa and the Olympians in their true form could prove fatal to a mortal, myths attest. As Hera says in Homer's epic the *Iliad*, 'the gods are dangerous when they appear in manifest form (*enargeis*)' (20.131). Many Greek myths warn of the dangers of looking at the divine. For example, Apollodorus' *Bibliotheca*, which was originally attributed to Apollodorus of Athens, born c. 180 BCE, but now understood to have been written by a different author c. second century CE, tells the tale of the mortal Actaeon who gazes upon the naked goddess Artemis and is subsequently turned into a stag (3.4.4, translated by J. G. Frazer).

Medusa's story is also found within *Bibliotheca*. In this mythical tale, Zeus takes the form of a stream of gold to father Perseus (the hero who shall later defeat Medusa) with the mortal princess Danae. This again provides evidence of a god manipulating vision during contact with a mortal, as Danae is denied the right to look at Zeus in his true form. Yet, sight within the myth of Medusa does not simply denote boundaries between humans and gods, nor is the Gorgon simply an apotropaic figure. Rather, I argue that sight within this myth also signifies Greek gender customs. According to the ancient texts of Greek physiognomists, mortal men were able to look more freely than their female counterparts, who preserved their modesty by bowing the head to avoid meeting the gaze of their male associates (Cairns 2005: 123–156). Medusa, with her powerful gaze, does not conform to such customs and thus Perseus, by beheading her and using her powers for his own means, claims the gaze for himself. The Gorgon's transgression of her gender role may explain why she was a particular threat to men, with only the Greek writer Pausanias' *Description of Greece* (c. 143–176 CE) explicitly describing a woman being turned to stone by Medusa's gaze (9.34.1-2). This chapter analyses the role of sight within the myth of Medusa, and will suggest that the Gorgon's petrifying gaze is threatening because it is owned by a woman.[1]

THE ANCIENT SOURCES

There are many pieces of ancient literary evidence that refer to Medusa. The Gorgon, not yet named as Medusa, is first mentioned in the Homeric epic the *Iliad* (the date of this work is disputed; Bernard Knox [1991] gives c. 725–675 BCE). Within this epic, the Gorgon is referenced in relation to armour and war, with her head imposed on the aegis of the goddess Athena (Homer *Il.* 5.741-742, translated by R. Lattimore) and also as a feature on Agamemnon's shield (*Il.* 11.36-37). The earliest surviving literary sources that introduce Medusa's subjugation by Perseus are Hesiod's (c. 700 BCE) *Theogony* (270-283) and *The Shield of Herakles* (220-237). The version of the myth that will be most familiar to the modern reader, however, derives from Apollodorus' *Bibliotheca* and the Roman poet Ovid's *Metamorphoses* (completed c. 8 CE). Both accounts draw on older sources, such as Hesiod and Pherecydes of Athens (fifth century BCE), to compile a more complete account of the adventures of Perseus. Medusa, however, is not the main focus of these narratives, rather she is a figure used to highlight Perseus' heroism.

1 Other sources mention groups of people being turned to stone by looking at the Gorgon, and we may assume this includes both men and women, for example, the Greek poet Pindar's *Pythian* 12 (c. 490 BCE) and the Roman poet Lucan's *Pharsalia* (9.651) (c. 61–65 CE).

Throughout the myth of Perseus and Medusa, there is an emphasis on the sense of sight and what can and cannot be seen. Indeed, sight is being manipulated at the beginning of the narrative, even before the arrival of Medusa and her petrifying gaze. As Apollodorus' account begins, it is the oracle which tells Acrisius, the king of Argos, that his daughter Danae will bear a son who will kill him. Fearing the prophecy, 'Acrisius built a brazen chamber underground and there guarded Danae' (Apollod. *Bibl.* 2.4.1). Zeus, however, is attracted to Danae and the underground chamber is not enough to deter the god from visiting the princess as a 'stream of gold' (*Bibl.* 2.4.1). Perseus is born and Acrisius locks both Danae and baby in a wooden chest, casting them out to sea. The mother and son survive and are washed up on the island of Seriphus. Sight is subtly manipulated here in a number of ways. It is the fearful Acrisius who removes his daughter from sight to prevent her from conceiving a son. Zeus, in contrast, is the light which enters Danae as a stream of gold, yet, when both mother and son are cast to sea, they are removed from sight *again* as they are removed from society (Mack 2002: 589). Sight is thus constantly being denied to Perseus at the beginning of his life, as is his patriarchal right to be successor to the throne.

It is when Perseus reaches adolescence that, in the true tradition of hero narrative, he must leave his home for adventure. Perseus must fetch Medusa's head to save his mother from Polydectes, the king of Seriphus, who wants Danae for himself. Medusa has two Gorgon sisters, Stheno and Euryale, but she alone is mortal and thus it is her head Perseus must claim. Since Medusa has the ability to petrify her victims through her gaze, Perseus must navigate a way to avoid the Gorgon's power to objectify. To do so, Perseus relies on the help of the gods Hermes and Athena who guide him to the Graeae, three eternally old women who are also sisters to the Gorgons (*Bibl.* 2.4.2). These hags have only one eye and a tooth between them. Here, Perseus manipulates the gaze by stealing the Graeae's only form of vision and, in an act that denies the women sight, situates the male in a dominant position. The hero only returns the eye after the sisters give him the location of nymphs who can supply Perseus with several objects to help him on his quest: 'these nymphs had in their possession winged sandals and the *kibisis*, which they say was a knapsack.... They also had the helmet of Hades' (*Bibl.* 2.4.2).

The gifts the nymphs bestow upon Perseus are all designed for his ability to control the gaze. The sandals, which give Perseus flight, make it difficult to see him, as does the helmet which makes the wearer invisible. Perseus controls who sees *him* while he is able to look freely: 'wearing it, he saw whom he pleased, but was not seen by others' (*Bibl.* 2.4.2). Using these gifts to access Medusa and her Gorgon sisters' lair, Perseus must now determine how he can defeat Medusa when he cannot look at her. In order to overcome this threat, Perseus looks at Medusa via her reflection on his shield. There are comparisons to be drawn here with another Greek myth where sight of one's reflection precedes death. Pausanias' *Description of Greece* (c. second century CE) tells the widely known myth of Narcissus who fell in love with his own reflection in a lake and subsequently 'died of love' (9.31.7–9). The myth of Medusa similarly contains the concept of reflection being a portent of death. Although Medusa is sleeping when her image is reflected on Perseus' shield, the mirror image still precedes her demise. Sight of one's reflection can be an omen of death, and this may shed light on why mirrors have repeatedly been found in Greek tombs (Seaford 1998: 105). There was also the idea within Greek thought that the mirror's image was the soul, providing another suggestion as to why they were thought to be connected with death. However, this magical function of the mirror seems to have disappeared after the late classical period (Melchior-Bonnet 2001: 102).

By Perseus gazing upon Medusa's image, roles have been reversed. The hero is now positioned as subject and is able to look at the Gorgon and objectify *her*. Perseus cuts off Medusa's head, the site of her power, and places it in his *kibisis*. The bag protects Perseus from the head of Medusa and, rather than destroying the Gorgon, he has claimed her power for himself. The *kibisis* thus serves as a veil which Perseus can use when he pleases to reveal and use the power of Medusa's gaze (Vernant 1991: 146). Perseus escapes the Gorgons' lair and runs away from Medusa's sisters by wearing the cap of Hades, which renders him invisible. The hero now owns Medusa's gaze. In this myth, power is held by the one who is positioned as subject; power *is* the gaze.

There are a number of occasions when Perseus uses Medusa's power for his own means. On his journey home, Perseus finds the beautiful, virginal Andromeda tied to rocks as a sacrifice to a sea monster. The hero saves the maiden and marries her, even though she was promised for marriage to Phineus. Consequently, Phineus plots his revenge against Perseus, but the hero discovers his scheme and, 'by showing the Gorgon turned him and his fellow conspirators at once into stone' (*Bibl.* 2.4.3). Furthermore, after returning to Seriphus, Perseus must show the Gorgon's head to save Danae, the hero:

[Perseus e]ntered the palace, where Polydectes had gathered his friends, and with averted face he showed the Gorgon's head; and all who beheld it were turned to stone, each in the attitude which he happened to have struck. (*Bibl.* 2.4.3)

The gaze itself does not appear problematic if it is owned by the male hero and not the uncontrolled female Gorgon. By adopting Medusa's gaze, I suggest that Perseus is restoring power to the male through the possession of sight. This theory is supplemented by ancient Greek literary evidence, discussed below, which praises the free (citizen) male's ability to look almost at will, while placing much firmer restrictions on women.

THE EYES AND THE GAZE IN ANCIENT GREEK SOCIETY

Douglas Cairns (2005) analyses the role and importance of the eyes in ancient Greek social interaction. Ancient physiognomists were particularly fascinated with the eyes and gave very specific and detailed accounts of inappropriate and appropriate forms of looking in the Greek world. The eyes of someone shameless, for example, would be unblinking (Adamantius 2.48, edition Foerster 1893: 413 used in Cairns 2005: 128). The brave male, in contrast, who exhibited 'a moist, gorgon's gaze, large eyes, not too wide open but not closed either, and a brow that is not too smooth or too furrowed' was taken with admiration according to the physiognomist Adamantius (2.44, edition Foerster 1893: 409–10 quoted in Cairns 2005: 128). The description 'gorgon's gaze' here is noteworthy. The Greek reads, '*blemma hygron gorgon*,' which means 'a moist, fierce gaze.' Thus 'gorgon' here is an adjective meaning 'fierce' or 'terrible' and this phrase would certainly have suggested the figure of Medusa, even though she is not mentioned. However, unlike the Gorgon's, the brave male's terrifying look is celebrated. Thus, can it be deduced that Medusa's gaze was only problematic because it was wielded by a *woman*?

Although there were very subtle differences between appropriate forms of looking, the free male's gaze was not subject to the harsh limitations dictated to women. Cairns considers the ideal female gaze and, in so doing, he acknowledges that the interpretations of the eyes by the physiognomists can only take a modern reader so far in understanding the gaze in regard to real social interactions. To gain a better understanding, Cairns suggests turning to 'human beings acting in plausible situations, i.e. to epic, drama and the novel' (2005: 128). Cairns finds that in his examination of these different platforms of Greek literature, the free male's gaze was far less restricted than the female's (2005: 133). As discussed above, Perseus, with the aid of the nymph's gifts and by using his shield's reflection, can look at whom he pleases, while he controls who looks at him. In terms of understanding the *female gaze*, however, this can be understood through the Greek term *aidos*. As classicist Helen King says, 'while in some contexts "shame" seems to be the best English translation of *aidos*, in others "modesty" would be the best fit' (2016: 195). Further, *aidos* is the 'acknowledgement of the status of others,' and, as the Greek woman had a lower social standing than the male, she was expected to have a lowered gaze (Cairns 2005: 134). This is evident in the following extract taken from Euripides' tragedy *Hecuba*, a tale set just after the Trojan war, where the title character says 'custom (*nomos*) forbids that a woman look into the eyes of men' (Eur. *Hec.* 974–975, used in Lloyd Llewellyn-Jones 2003: 165, who also suggests that veiling was another way the Greek woman demonstrated *aidos*). Therefore, '*aidos* in the eyes' is an expression often attributed to women in Greek myth in reference to her downcast gaze signalling that she was in the company of a person of higher status (Cairns 2005: 134). An example is the Choice of Heracles in Xenophon's *Memorabilia* where Arete, a female personification of Virtue, can be read as having *aidos* in the eyes:

> For adornment her body had purity, her eyes modesty, her bearing moderation, and she had white clothing. The other had been fed to the point of being fleshy and soft. She was prettied up so that her complexion seemed to appear whiter and rosier than its reality, and so that her bearing seemed straighter than its nature. Her eyes were wide open, and she was wearing the clothes in which her bloom would be most conspicuous. She looked down at herself frequently, looked around to see if anyone else was looking at her, and frequently looked at her own shadow. (Xen. *Mem.* 2.1.22, translated by A. L. Bonnette)

The 'other' here is Kakia, Vice. The two women are contrasted with each other. Whereas Arete's eyes are 'modest,' Kakia's eyes are 'wide open.' The eyes of a woman who does not lower her gaze were 'taken by physiognomists as a sign that she is a prostitute' (Pseudo-Polemo 81, edition Foerster 1893: 430 and Jesus Siracides 26.9, edition Foerster 1893: 272 taken from Cairns 2005: 134). If the physiognomists interpreted the upward female gaze as being indicative that she was a prostitute, can Medusa be read as an overtly sexual woman, with her ability to gaze at men and stupefy them? I would argue, using Jean-Pierre Vernant, that Medusa *steals* the male gaze by reflecting it back onto her onlooker (Vernant 1991: 137). This situates Medusa in the male's position as *subject*, whereas her victim has become a stone *object* devoid of sight.

For the ancient Greeks, sight signified the distinction between the superior and the inferior. Just as respectable women were modest in the presence of men, so the gods controlled who gazed at their true form because of their vast superiority. Social boundaries, as well as the boundary between the divine and the mortal, are distinguished through looking and thus we can infer that Medusa's objectifying gaze signifies her transgression from the socially desired behaviour of the modest woman and situates her in more of a masculine role. In the next section, I shall further argue that Medusa takes a typically male position and that this is through her ability to *create*.

SIGHT AS TOUCH

Interestingly, within the ancient literature there is a suggestion that sight was aligned with the sense of touch. As classicist Shadi Bartsch says:

> almost all the ancient schools of thought about optics, from the atomists to Plato, Euclid, and Ptolemy, put an emphasis on the tactile nature of sight, and several of them talk specifically in terms of penetration and touching in language that is literal, not metaphorical. (Bartsch 2014: 59)

An example of such tactile descriptions is found in Plato's *Timaeus* (c. 360 BCE): 'this happens wherever the internal fire strikes and presses against an external object it has connected with' (45c, translated by D. J. Zeyl). According to Plato, it is the 'internal fire' from the eyes that momentarily integrates with daylight in order to 'form a body that touches (*ephaptetoi*) objects at a distance' (Bartsch 2014: 63). This can be aligned with Medusa. It is Medusa's sight that causes change in her victims, turning them into objects. To objectify is to demote something, often by looking at it, to the position of an object. Yet in Medusa's case she has literally turned that something *into* an object. With her victims turned into lifeless statues, Medusa is positioned as a sculptor, a creator of images.

Creating through touch is prominent in the myth of Pygmalion, who creates sculptures. The tale was originally found in Philostephanus of

Cyrene's work *De Cypro* (thought to have been written during the Hellenistic period c. third century BCE), where Pygmalion of Cyprus falls in love with a cult statue of the goddess Aphrodite (Miller 1990: 205). This work has since been lost but had a profound influence on the version of the myth in *Metamorphoses*, a collection of largely Greek myths regarding the theme of transformation, reworked and embellished by the Roman poet Ovid. In Ovid's version, Pygmalion becomes the sculptor with Venus (Aphrodite) no longer the statue. Rather, in this version, the goddess gives life to Pygmalion's ivory creation of a woman. The gods transforming mortals into objects, which here appears in reverse, is a recurring theme within Ovid's epic.

It is interesting that the myths of Medusa and Pygmalion are found within *Metamorphoses*, as these figures create statues by sight and touch respectively. Thus, I suggest that the concept of sight being tactile in nature, as argued by earlier Greek thought, becomes an actuality in this later Roman work *because* Medusa is presented as a sculptor. I shall first analyse the myth of Pygmalion as it is found in Ovid (*Met.* 10.243–297) before presenting a correlation with Medusa.

The myth of Pygmalion begins with the sculptor creating an ivory figure of a beautiful woman whom he falls in love with. There is a heavy, sensual focus on the way Pygmalion caresses this statue, using his hands to feel the inanimate girl he created:

> His heart desired the body he had formed.
> With many a touch he tries it – is it flesh
> Or ivory? Not ivory still, he's sure!
> Kisses he gives and thinks they are returned;
> He speaks to it, caresses it, believes
> The firm new flesh beneath his fingers yields,
> And fears the limbs may darken with a bruise.
> (*Met.* 10.254–258)

The tactile nature of the narrative is a reminder that it is Pygmalion who has created the girl with his own hands and that he has authority over her. As art historian Victor Stoichita says in *The Pygmalion Effect*, '"to touch the work" is to demote it to the status of an object' (2008: 1). Pygmalion, in his role as sculptor, can manipulate the female image and as he gazes upon her body and touches her, she cannot reciprocate.

There is a suggestion made by Ovid that this statue is not simply an ivory carving, with the line 'such art his art concealed' (*Met.* 10.252). As

Edward. J. Kenney, in his accompanying notes to *Metamorphoses*, says, 'the ancients were firmly convinced of the virtues of representational art' and here Ovid reveals that Pygmalion's girl is not simply an imitation (Ovid 2008: 434). This has led art historian Caroline van Eck to read Medusa as Pygmalion's 'dark double,' an 'anti-Pygmalion, petrifying where the sculptor animates' (2016: 6–7). Van Eck refers to Ovid's description of Medusa's lair which draws similarities with a garden filled with ornamental statues (2016: 7):

> Of ruined woods he reached the Gorgons' land
> And everywhere in fields and by the road
> He saw the shapes of men and beasts, all changed
> To stone by glancing at Medusa's face.
> (*Met.* 4.780–781)

Similarly, when Perseus uses the Gorgon's power against Phineus and the rest of his assailants, Ovid describes the victims as 'marble' (*Met.* 5.198–199).

Whereas Medusa turns her victims into statues, it is Pygmalion who gives the statue *life*. Pygmalion wishes and wills his statue to be real but dares not ask this from the goddess Venus when he prays at her altar. The goddess, however, knows Pygmalion's true desire and she grants him his wish:

> And he went home, home to his heart's delight,
> And kissed her as she lay, and she seemed warm;
> Again he kissed her and with marvelling touch
> Caressed her breast; beneath his touch the flesh
> Grew soft, its ivory hardness vanishing....
> (*Met.* 10.280–284)

Pygmalion fears that this is an illusion so he touches her 'again and again' (*Met.* 10.288). Pygmalion objectifies the statue with his touch and his gaze and, when the image comes to life, the girl blushes at his kisses and 'shyly' raises her eyes (*Met.* 10.293). 'Shyly' serves as a contrast between the gaze of Pygmalion and his statue, with the girl maintaining a modest pose, typical of the female displaying the notion of *aidos*, discussed above. If sight and touch are aligned, then Medusa poses a double threat. Her ability to objectify, both figuratively and literally, I suggest, fully positions her in an active, and thus male, position. The Gorgon seems to truly embody chaos in the ancient world because of her transgression of gender boundaries.

MEDUSA'S IMAGE: SEEING THE UNSEEABLE

Medusa is not just found in literary examples from the ancient world. Medusa's eyes that could famously turn victims to stone led to her position as an apotropaic icon. According to Albert. M. Potts' research regarding the significance of the eye as a symbol, 'apotropaic' derives from 'the Greek *apo* (away from) and *trope* (turn)' (1982: 26). An apotropaic device has the ability to turn evil away, just as individuals would turn away from Medusa to avoid her gaze. This sheds light on why the Gorgon is found, either full-bodied or simply her head (the gorgoneion), on many discovered temples dedicated to various Olympian deities across the Greek world.

The Temple of Artemis, Corfu (c. 580 BCE) is a particularly excellent example of the Gorgon being a significant figure on a Greek temple. Here, Medusa is featured on the pediment and is shown in profile alongside her children, Chrysaor and Pegasus, with a lion on either side (lions are also apotropaic in the ancient Greek World, see A. David Napier's *Masks, Transformation, and Paradox* [1986: 108]). Interestingly, Medusa, Chrysaor and the lions have their heads turned to directly meet the gaze of any visitor to the temple. Medusa stands at an imposing height of around three metres and her most prominent feature appears to be her eyes, which bulge from her head (Stansbury-O'Donnell 2015: 184). This example is made from stone but on the Temple of Athena, Syracuse (c. 575–550 BCE) the Gorgon is fashioned from terracotta. Here, she would have been found either on the acroterion or pediment and with brightly coloured 'red tongue and red and black pupils in her eyes' (Holloway 1991: 80). The focus in these examples is quite clearly on sight, with Medusa looking at visitors and passersby. Medusa on the Temple of Athena is shown full-bodied with Pegasus. Like the Temple of Artemis in Corfu, this depiction does not make narrative sense, as Stansbury-O'Donnell notes (2015: 185). Chrysaor and Pegasus are born after Perseus has decapitated Medusa, yet the Gorgon stands side-by-side with her children, her head attached to her body. Thus, rather than making narrative sense, the Gorgon when found on prominent locations such as the antefix or pediment of a temple was simply used for her apotropaic power.

The Gorgon, as a popular apotropaic image, was not limited to protecting temples. Her image is found everywhere in the Greek world, from roof tiles to symposium cups. Rainer Mack (2002) studies the gorgoneion (which, as noted above, was simply the image of the Gorgon's head) during the period from the early seventh to late fifth century BCE, when focus was on the Gorgon's eyes which were large and 'stared out from the picture field in a hypnotic manner, encircled by folds of flesh and a ring of wild hair' (Mack 2002: 572). Mack also argues that the Gorgon was an apotropaic figure and cites Homer as evidence, 'thereon is set the head of the grim gigantic Gorgon, a thing of fear and horror' (*Il.* 5.741–742). Homer does not directly describe the Gorgon, later known as Medusa, but rather describes the terror she incites in others. This is because Homer is describing the *unseeable* as the viewer is 'turned away' from the image, suggesting the Gorgon's capability to deflect the evil eye as an apotropaic device (Mack 2002: 573, 576).

It is odd, however, that the gorgoneion was repeatedly made and dispersed for consumption and thus produced not just to ward off the evil eye, but to be looked *at* (Mack 2002: 574). It is also questionable whether sight of the Gorgon would have terrified viewers, because they were in contact with her image so often. Mack suggests that the purpose of Medusa's image is thus more complex than her simply being an apotropaic icon. As in the myth when Perseus looks at Medusa through the reflection on his shield, Medusa loses her subjectivity when the viewer gazes at her image. The viewer is thus placed in the dominant Perseus position with Medusa's image posing a 'staged threat,' for she symbolises a danger which has already been conquered by Perseus: 'when image-makers and image-viewers "defeated" the gaze of Medusa, they were defeating a phantom, for they were only doing what Perseus had already done' (Mack 2002: 588). Mack thus argues that in nearly all images of Medusa, Perseus' presence is suggested. The gorgoneion suggests that she has already been decapitated and defeated by Perseus. Even in cases when Medusa's full body is depicted, with her head attached, Perseus' presence is usually alluded to. For example, on the Temple of Artemis in Corfu, discussed above, Medusa is shown with Chrysaor and Pegasus, the children she conceived with Poseidon. According to the ancient texts, Medusa's children are born after her death, of the blood spilled from her beheading by Perseus, and thus the hero's presence is still felt here. Unlike Stansbury-O'Donnell (above), Mack argues that the image can only be understood in relation to the myth because Perseus' subjugation of the Gorgon is usually, if not always, insinuated. Therefore, when the viewer looks at the gorgoneion, he or she becomes an 'image-maker' like Perseus and 'in the simple act of viewing the image…re-enact[s] his heroic triumph over the monster' (Mack 2002: 593).

Rather than the gorgoneion being simply apotropaic, it also represents Perseus' heroism. It signifies Perseus' reclamation of the gaze in two ways. First, Perseus is able to look at Medusa's head on his shield via reflection, thus subjugating the Gorgon by reducing her to an object and placing himself as subject. Second, Perseus steals Medusa's head and uses it for his own means. This transfer of power, which situates Perseus in the dominant viewing position, is best encapsulated in the image on an Attic red-figure *pelike* (Pan Painter, c. 480 used in Mack 2002: 587). Perseus is shown with his body front-facing, yet his head is turned to the side, looking away from the decapitated Gorgon's head he holds in his hand. Medusa is shown with gaping mouth and is facing the viewer. Here, the Pan Painter is demonstrating that Perseus is in full possession of Medusa's gaze, as if Perseus is looking *through* Medusa's eyes (Mack 2002: 598).

The gorgoneion, when depicted on certain items, also allows the user to manipulate and utilise her gaze, just as Perseus does. Agamemnon, for example, in Homer's *Iliad* wears the gorgoneion on his shield which looks out onto his enemies. With Agamemnon behind the shield, Medusa's face becomes a mask and thus the hero appropriates Medusa's gaze for himself. Rather than the Gorgon being simply a threat to Agamemnon's enemies, her head represents Agamemnon as a hero. As the gorgoneion is already decapitated, the image can be understood in relation to the myth and Perseus' subjugation of Medusa. It is Perseus' shield after all where the hero is able to look at Medusa's image. Therefore, Agamemnon is situated as Perseus, an image-maker who is in a dominant viewing position. Again, power is aligned with the gaze. Similarly, the symposiast at the symposium also manipulated Medusa's gaze for himself. The drinking cups used by symposiasts often featured the Gorgon's head on the outside of the cup and on the inside at the base. Thus, when the symposiast lifted his cup to drink, the Gorgon's image and gaze would become his own as a mask, as the outside image looked out onto the room (Mack 2002: 578). Further, as the symposiast finished his wine, the gorgoneion image at the bottom of the cup would be revealed to him. This was not terrifying but would rather act as the symposiast's reflection, his mirror-other, 'whose gaze calls attention to your own' (Mack 2002: 578). Both engagements with the gorgoneion reaffirm the symposiast as the subject of the gaze. Therefore, the '(mythological discourse) articulates a threat that the other (imaging) instantiates and, in the same manoeuvre, overcomes' (Mack 2002: 578). The symposium was a male-only drinking party and, like the Gorgon's image on the shield, fully aligns masculinity with the dominant viewing position.

Mack thus argues that the myth of Perseus and Medusa provides an 'aetiology of the gaze' (2002: 589). As has been discussed earlier in this chapter, Perseus, prior to claiming Medusa's head, is consistently denied sight.

By Perseus stealing the gaze from Medusa, the myth acts as an aetiological story of the male's claim, or right, to look. Therefore, the gorgoneion encapsulates 'the aetiological argument of the legend with an efficiency not possible in narrative discourse' (Mack 2002: 593). Thus, Medusa is more than simply an apotropaic icon. Medusa is a female whose possession of the gaze represents disorder and chaos. Perseus must claim the gaze for himself to signify his authority and patriarchal right to look freely and the female is consequently reduced to being the object of the male's gaze in a restoration of Greek gender ideals.

Ann Suter takes the gendered elements of the Medusa myth and the Gorgon's gaze further, although, unlike Mack, she argues that this is found only in the literature and not on 'architectural antefixes' (2015: 30). For Suter, Medusa's head is comparable to the *anasyrma*, the exposure of the female genitals. The *anasyrma* in ancient Greek myth is performed by the mortal nurse Baubo, who revealed her genitalia to liven the distraught goddess Demeter when her daughter Persephone had been abducted by Hades. This tale further highlights the importance of sight between mortal and divine relationships, with Baubo's act bringing the goddess brief relief from her anguish. The sight of the female genitals has a strikingly different effect when compared with the exposure of the male's. Whereas the male's genitals are associated with crudeness, female genitalia are, 'a movement, a gesture of revelation that is unexpected' and it is in this 'revelation' of the hidden that its powers lie (Suter 2015: 21). The *anasyrma* and Medusa's head are similar in that they both have largely positive effects on women, yet are detrimental to men. The *anasyrma* as used by Baubo in the example provided above gives comfort to a goddess who is battling against a *male* god. Similarly, Medusa also affects women who gaze upon her *positively* as both Medusa and the *anasyrma* are used to enhance female fertility. For example, the priestess of Athena shakes her aegis, which bears the image of the gorgoneion, 'at newly married Athenian wives,' which was taken as a method for enhancing the fertility of a new wife (Suter 2015: 23). Interestingly, there is only one known case from ancient myth where a woman is explicitly said to turn to stone via the Gorgon's gaze. The account is provided by Pausanias, who tells the tale of a Boeotian priestess, Iodama:

> The following tale, too, is told. Iodama, who served the goddess as priestess, entered the precinct by night, where there appeared to her Athena, upon whose tunic was worked the head of Medusa the Gorgon. When Iodama saw it, she was turned to stone. (Pausanias *Description of Greece,* 9.34.2, translated by W. H. S. Jones)

In contrast to the apparent beneficial effects Medusa and the *anasyrma* can have on the female spectator, catching sight of Medusa or the gesture of the *anasyrma* can have harmful effects when viewed by a male. Helen King in *The One-Sex Body on Trial* (2016) discusses war stories from the ancient world where women perform the *anasyrma* to shame their husbands who have returned from battle because of cowardice. One case is provided by Plutarch in his *Virtues of Women*, where the *anasyrma* is performed by the Persian women to convince their men to return to war (5.246a). These women, while lifting their garments to reveal their genitals, verbally invite their husbands to return to the wombs from which they were born (King 2016: 208). Thus, the *anasyrma* is more than just the revealing of the female genitals, it also suggests the womb (King 2016: 208). Like Baubo, these are mature women and King only mentions one case when the *anasyrma* is performed by a virgin. Unlike Baubo, however, this act is not intended to be humorous. The women who display their genitals do so in order to 'evoke in the male audience a feeling of *aidos* or of *aischyne*' (King 2016: 209). It was a way of shaming men back into their role as warriors while highlighting, by invoking the womb, that a woman's duty was to give birth; thus these women were re-establishing gender roles through the use of the *anasyrma* (King 2016: 209).

There are examples of the *anasyrma* being performed for other purposes. There is the abnormal case from Egypt where Hathor, the King Ra's daughter, performs an *anasyrma* to make her father happy (Suter 2015: 27 using Blackledge 2004: 18 who attributes the source to 'a papyrus from 1160 BCE recalling the myth'). Hathor's *anasyrma* works, thus showing that this act can be performed for a number of purposes, carrying out 'the will of the woman performing it' (Suter 2015: 27).

Significantly, it is *sight* which activates the power of both the *anasyrma* and Medusa, and it is the gender of the spectator that determines the effect. Medusa's alignment with the *anasyrma* goes further: it can be suggested that Medusa was aligned with female genitalia in the ancient world. Suter gives the example of a bronze disc which depicts Medusa with her genitals visible, found in the *LIMC* (1988: 4.1, 337, no. 87). Interestingly, during the early twentieth century, psychoanalyst Sigmund Freud also connected Medusa's head with the female genitals. According to Freud's essay 'Medusa's Head' (1922), Medusa is a symbol of castration anxiety and represents the young male's first *sight* of the mother's vagina. The young boy is attracted to his mother but after viewing her genitalia, which is different from his own, assumes that the father has castrated her and will do the same to him if he does not displace his affection for her onto another, more suitable, woman. Freud took Medusa's snake hair to be symbolic of the female pubic hair. To overcome this anxiety, the male fetishises Medusa, viewing her snakes as multiple phalluses which 'serve as a mitigation of the horror, for they replace the penis, the absence of which is the cause of the horror' (Freud 1922: 85). Medusa's glare also makes the male 'stiff with terror,' a euphemism for an erection and a reminder that he is still in possession of his own penis (Freud 1922: 85). Medusa's gaze is thus a source of both horror and pleasure for the male. By reducing the female to purely a fetish, the young boy resolves his fear of the woman who 'frightens and repels because she is castrated' (Freud 1922: 85). Perseus, then, is able to resolve his anxiety by looking at Medusa via her reflection on his shield which enables him to be situated in a superior viewing position, allowing him to decapitate the Gorgon. By subjecting the Gorgon to his gaze and overcoming her threat, Perseus can symbolically enter manhood by marrying the virginal and non-threatening Andromeda. Just as Freud argued that the sight of the female genitalia was terrifying for the male, Suter argues that the gender of the *viewer* is critical for understanding Medusa's effect. For the female spectator, Medusa seems to pose little danger.

Medusa's harmful effect on men is evident in examples outside of the Perseus myth. In Homer, Medusa is described as either being on Athena's aegis or on Agamemnon's shield. Thus, she is used on the battlefield against *men*. It is also evident in the following excerpt from the *Odyssey* where the protagonist Odysseus worries that 'Persephone might send forth upon me from out the house of Hades the head of the Gorgon, that awful monster' (11.634–235, translated by A. T. Murray). The different effects of Medusa's gaze based on the gender of the viewer are also apparent in Attic tragedy. Suter gives two examples from Euripides' plays where the effects of the Gorgon's gaze on women and men are generally taken as 'protective' and 'threatening' respectively (Suter 2015: 31). In *Ion*, Medusa's image is sewn by Creusa onto her son, Ion's, baby clothes (1413–1421). It is through the image of the gorgoneion that Ion recognises his mother later in life just as he is about to kill her. That the image was placed on the clothing of a baby also signifies Medusa's association with fertility. In contrast, in Euripides' *Elektra* (1218–1221), Orestes takes the role of Perseus when he kills his mother and must cover his face to avoid the gaze of Clytemnestra (who is positioned as Medusa) (Suter 2015: 31). Suter concludes that the different effects of Medusa relate to man and woman's different positions in society. Whereas the male protects the home by fighting, the female reproduces to ensure society's continuity (Suter 2015: 33). However, based on the material discussed within this chapter, I would argue that the suggestion of Medusa posing more of a threat to *men* is more likely explained by her gaze that upsets and disrupts male dominance.

CONCLUSION

As a final thought, I propose that modern feminist film theory can be used to further extrapolate ideas regarding the gaze and gender in ancient Greece. Medusa's gaze renders her a very complex character. Sight within this myth signifies the boundary between life and death, the mortal and the divine, and she is an apotropaic icon as well. However, I have argued that Medusa's gaze also marks her transgression of Greek gender boundaries, for to look freely was a male attribute. The gaze as *male* is an argument also made in feminist film theory. Laura Mulvey, for example, uses Freud's castration theory in her seminal essay 'Visual Pleasure and Narrative Cinema' (1975) to suggest that the female in cinema does not look but is to be looked *at* as the object of the 'male gaze'. Like Mulvey, French feminist Luce Irigaray argues that woman is denied sight, suggesting that she is more closely aligned with the sense of touch, 'for her genitals are formed of two lips in continuous contact' (1977b: 24). Medusa's sight, as has been discussed, can be read as a form of touch and offers an interesting point for discussion.

Teresa de Lauretis (1984) suggests that the female is the object of the gaze in cinema and reads the cinema screen as Perseus' shield, which repeatedly displays to the spectator the hero's subjugation of powerful women. This has interesting parallels with the gorgoneion, above, which enables the viewer to take Perseus' role and repeatedly objectify and defeat the Gorgon. Thus, the powerful woman in cinema, like Medusa, is *trapped* within this hero's narrative. Yet, there is room for reading Medusa as a subversive figure. If woman is object to the male gaze, then Medusa subverts this notion by reflecting the male's gaze back onto his self in a fatal act of petrification; she looks *back*. These are simply suggestions for areas of further research but it does become clearer, by using feminist film theory, that Medusa may have posed such a threat to men because she was not simply an object but a woman *who dared to look*.

BIBLIOGRAPHY

Primary Sources

Apollodorus. (2003) *The Library*. Translated by J. G. Frazer. New York and London: Routledge.
Homer. (1998) *Odyssey*. Translated by A. T. Murray. Second edition. Cambridge, Massachusetts: Harvard University Press.
Homer. (2003) *The Iliad*. Translated by R. Lattimore. New York and London: Routledge.
Ovid. (2008) *Metamorphoses*. Translated by A. D. Melville. Oxford: Oxford University Press.
Plato. (2000) *Timaeus*. Translated by D. J. Zeyl. Indianapolis: Hackett.
Pausanias. (2014) *Description of Greece*. Translated by W. H. S. Jones. eBook: Delphi Classics.
Xenophon. (2001) *Memorabilia*. Translated by A. L. Bonnette. Ithaca and London: Cornell University Press.

Secondary Sources

Bartsch, S. (2014) *The Mirror of the Self: Sexuality, Self-Knowledge, and the Gaze in the Early Roman Empire*. Chicago and London: University of Chicago Press.
Blackledge, C. (2004) *The Story of V: A Natural History of Female Sexuality*. New Jersey: Rutgers University Press.
Blundell, S. (1995) *Women in Ancient Greece*. Cambridge, MA: Harvard University Press.
Bowers, S. R. (1990) 'Medusa and the Female Gaze,' *NWSA Journal*, 2(2), 217–235. Available at: http://www.jstor.org/stable/4316018 [accessed on 27 February 2019].
Bredekamp, H. (2018) *Image Acts: A Systematic Approach to Visual Agency* (translated by E. Clegg). Berlin: De Gruyter. https://doi.org/10.1515/9783110548570
Cairns, D. (2005) 'Bullish Looks and Sidelong Glances: Social Interaction and the Eyes in Ancient Greek Culture,' in Cairns, D. (ed.), *Body Language in the Greek and Roman Worlds*. Swansea: The Classical Press of Wales, pp. 123–156. https://doi.org/10.2307/j.ctvvn97x.10
Cixous, H. (1975) 'The Laugh of Medusa' (translated by K. Cohen and P. Cohen), in Garber, M. and Vickers, N. J. (eds.), *The Medusa Reader* (2003). New York and London: Routledge, pp. 133–134. https://doi.org/10.1007/978-1-349-14428-0_21
De Lauretis, T. (1984) *Alice Doesn't: Feminism, Semiotics, Cinema*. Indianapolis: Indiana University Press. https://doi.org/10.1007/978-1-349-17495-9
Freud, S. (1922) 'Medusa's Head,' in Garber, M. and Vickers, N. J. (eds.), *The Medusa Reader* (2003). New York and London: Routledge, pp. 84–85.
Holloway, R. R. (1991) *The Archaeology of Ancient Sicily*. London: Routledge.
Irigaray, L. (1977a) 'Women's Exile' (translated by C. Venn), *Ideology and Consciousness*, 1, 62–76.
Irigaray, L. (1977b) *This Sex Which is Not One* (translated by C. Porter and C. Burke) (1985). New York: Cornell University Press. https://doi.org/10.1007/978-1-349-14428-0_22

Keuls, E. C. (1993) *The Reign of the Phallus: Sexual Politics in Ancient Athens*. Berkeley: University of California Press.

King, H. (1998) *Hippocrates' Woman: Reading the Female Body in Ancient Greece*. New York and London: Routledge.

King, H. (2016) *The One-Sex Body on Trial: The Classical and Early Modern Evidence*. Oxford: Routledge. https://doi.org/10.4324/9781315555027

Knox, B. (1991) 'Introduction,' in Homer, *The Iliad* (translated by R. Fagles). New York: Penguin, pp. 3–64.

Leeming, D. (2013) *Medusa: In the Mirror of Time*. London: Reaktion Books.

Lewis, D. B. (2015) *The Mythology of Medusa: A Complete Reference*. CreateSpace Independent Publishing Platform.

Llewellyn-Jones, L. (2003) *Aphrodite's Tortoise: The Veiled Woman of Ancient Greece*. Swansea: The Classical Press of Wales.

Lijun, M. (2015) *Human and Horses – Ancient Art* [online]. Available at: https://ancientart.as.ua.edu/human-and-horses/ [accessed on 12 July 2018].

LIMC (1988) *Lexicon Iconographicum Mythologiae Classicae*. Zurich: Artemis.

Mack, R. (2002). 'Facing Down Medusa (An Aetiology of the Gaze),' *Art History*, 25(5), 571–604. https://doi.org/10.1111/1467-8365.00346

Melchior-Bonnet, S. (2001) *The Mirror: A History* (translated by K. H. Jewett). New York and London: Routledge.

Miller, J. M. (1990) 'Some Versions of Pygmalion,' in Martindale, C., *Ovid Renewed: Ovidian Influences on Literature and Art from the Middle Ages to the Twentieth Century*. Cambridge: Cambridge University Press, pp. 205–214.

Mulvey, L. (1975) 'Visual Pleasure and Narrative Cinema,' in Kaplan, E. A. (ed.), *Feminism and Film*. Oxford: Oxford University Press, pp. 34–47. https://doi.org/10.1007/978-1-349-14428-0_27

Mulvey, L. (1981) 'Afterthoughts on "Visual Pleasure and Narrative Cinema" Inspired by King Vidor's Duel in the Sun (1946),' in Mulvey, L., *Visual and Other Pleasures* (1989). New York: Palgrave, pp. 29–38. https://doi.org/10.1007/978-1-349-19798-9_4

Musgrove, M. W. (2000) *The Student's Ovid: Selections from the Metamorphoses*. Oklahoma: University of Oklahoma Press.

Napier, A. D. (1986) *Masks, Transformation, and Paradox*. Los Angeles: University of California Press.

Ogden, D. (2008) *Perseus*. Oxford: Routledge. https://doi.org/10.4324/9780203932131

Platt, V. (2016) 'Sight and the Gods: On the Desire to See Naked Nymphs,' in Squire, M. (ed.), *Sight and the Ancient Senses*. London and New York: Routledge, pp. 161–179.

Pollock, G. (2006) 'Beyond Oedipus: Feminist Thought, Psychoanalysis, and Mythical Figurations of the Feminine,' in Zajko, V. and Leonard, M. (eds.), *Laughing with Medusa: Classical Myth and Feminist Thought*. New York: Oxford University Press, pp. 67–120.

Potts, A. M. (1982) *The World's Eye*. Kentucky: The University Press of Kentucky.

Seaford, R. (1998) 'In the Mirror of Dionysos,' in Blundell, S. and Williamson, M. (eds.), *The Sacred and the Feminine in Ancient Greece*. London and New York: Routledge, pp. 101–117.

Stansbury-O'Donnell, M, D. (2015) *A History of Greek Art*. Oxford: Wiley.

Stoichita, V. I. (2008) *The Pygmalion Effect: From Ovid to Hitchcock* (translated by A. Anderson). Chicago and London: University of Chicago Press.
Suter, A. (2015) 'The Anasyrma: Baubo, Medusa, and the Gendering of Obscenity,' in Dutsch, D. and Suter, A. (eds.), *Ancient Obscenities: Their Nature and Use in the Ancient Greek and Roman Worlds*. Michigan: University of Michigan Press, pp. 21–43.
Van Eck, C. (2015) *Art, Agency and Living Presence: From the Animated Image to the Excessive Object*. Boston: De Gruyter. https://doi.org/10.1515/9783110345568
Van Eck, C. (2016) 'The Petrifying Gaze of Medusa: Ambivalence, *Ekplexis*, and the Sublime,' *Journal of Historians of Netherlandish Art*, 8(2), Summer, 1–22. Available at: http://www.jhna.org/index.php/vol-8-2-2016/336-caroline-van-eck [accessed on 27 February 2019]. https://doi.org/10.5092/jhna.2016.8.2.3
Vernant, J. (1991) 'Death in the Eyes: Gorgo, Figure of the Other' and 'In the Mirror of Medusa,' in Zeitlin, F. (ed.), *Mortals and Immortals: Collected Essays*. New Jersey: Princeton University Press, pp. 111–138 and 141–150 respectively.
Wilk, S, R. (2000) *Medusa: Solving the Mystery of the Gorgon*. New York: Oxford University Press.

Gina Bevan is a current PhD student at Cardiff University. Her thesis, 'The Ambivalence of Medusa: Female Use of the Gorgon in Popular Culture from the 1980s to the Present' is an interdisciplinary work which combines the topics of religion, ancient history and gender. Gina has presented her PhD research at a number of conferences, including a piece which explored rap artist Azealia Banks' use of Medusa in her 'Ice Princess' music video. It appears that Banks may be using the Gorgon as a symbol of black female experience, and Gina's findings were presented at the 2017 Classical Antiquity and Memory conference, University of Bonn and the 2017 UWICAH conference, University of Wales. Gina also enjoys teaching and she is currently a mentor for The Brilliant Club, a charity which seeks to increase the number of talented but less fortunate students applying to highly selective universities.

Chapter 6

'A Power Invisible': How Somnambulists' Blindness Reflected Debate on the Existence of the Soul

MARTINA BARTLETT

> Many somnambulists have been known to see in complete darkness, while their eyes, besides, were proved to be insensible to the stimulus of light. (Colquhoun 1845: 19)

Imagine the scene: a young girl of about twelve years old, eyes closed and blindfolded, and yet able to recognise colours and patterns held up before her, as well as cut figures out of paper (Colquhoun 1845 [1805]: 47). This is just one of the examples Bremen physician Arnold Wienholt (1749–1804) gave near the beginning of his work, *Seven Lectures on Somnambulism*, written in German, of cases where sufferers of sleep disorders and conditions affecting the nervous system demonstrated the use of sight even when, physically, they should not be able to see. Wienholt's work was published posthumously in 1805 and translated into English by J. C. Colquhoun (1803–1870) in 1845 when there was a revival of interest in trance states such as that of somnambulism.[1]

Wienholt's series of lectures begins with the recognition of changes in philosophy, which according to Colquhoun's footnote, is directly related

---

1 Wienholt's translator, J. C. Colquhoun added a substantial preface, introduction and appendix, and quotes have been taken from these. In order to identify quotes taken from Wienholt's lectures as opposed to quotes from Colquhoun's additions, the original publication date has been added in square brackets to text citations, [1805].

to the work of philosopher Immanuel Kant. In short, Wienholt noted that philosophy questioned human cognitive faculties, and for him this seemed a welcome challenge to intellectual certainty. However, in Wienholt's opinion, the inquiry fell short, and did not extend to what he described as *'empirical psychology'* (Colquhoun 1845: 38, original italics). Wienholt described how philosophers could recognise the material body and its interconnectedness with what he called a 'transcendent something' and see that the physical systems of the body were essential to the soul 'in the due exercise of its functions' (1845: 39), but would not admit a lack of knowledge. 'He [the philosopher] does not, or will not see, that this compound being, so far as relates to the functions of the supersensible principle, lies beyond the sphere of his knowledge' (1845: 39). In brief, Wienholt suggested that philosophers only considered the physical and metaphysical body through its mechanical systems. For Wienholt the condition of somnambulism, at this time in the late eighteenth and early nineteenth century, resisted true explanation, specifically the phenomenon wherein somnambulists seemed to see without using their eyes.

The end of the eighteenth century saw paradigmatic shifts across Europe, with new perspectives forged in the fires of revolution. Natural philosophy began developing into more defined scientific disciplines, although this was to take the better part of the nineteenth century. Scientific enquiries confirmed for philosophers and physicians of a materialist viewpoint that nature in general, and human beings in particular, were mechanical systems. However, despite rationalist thinking, which sought material explanations for all aspects of human existence, some metaphysical, or seemingly supernatural, phenomena resisted explanation and could not be easily dismissed as belonging to an outmoded paradigm (see Thomas 1991: 767–800).

Throughout the eighteenth century there were many changes in ideas about how the organic body functioned, for example the importance of blood and blood vessels, the spinal cord and involuntary actions, and the effect of the nervous system on health and disease. A highly rational approach to the organic world gave rise to fears that human beings were mechanical creatures. The creation of automata, such as Jacques Vaucanson's digesting duck, which was displayed in a Parisian exhibition in 1738, demonstrated human creativity of the Enlightenment, and also became a physical embodiment of the fears that humans might be soulless automata. Luigi Galvani (1737–1798) investigated 'animal electricity' and artificially stimulated nerve-endings (for example those of frog's legs) and produced involuntary actions.[2] The discovery that non-human organisms had similar systems to humans added to the questions around the nature of human life.

Interest in electricity and its potential also led, in part, to enhanced understanding of the nervous system. At the same time, hypotheses for the seat of that vital principle, or life force, were fiercely debated; surgeon John Hunter favouring the blood and the circulatory system, others preferring the nervous system (Bynum 2006: 14). The relationship with the divine soul added another layer of complexity to the arguments. Scottish physician William Cullen (1710–1790), was able to integrate the systems of the human body with the metaphysical. Cullen lectured on the nervous system, stressing that although its mechanisms and that of the brain could be observed, they could not be explained without the immaterial soul, which he said was the source of 'nervous power, or energy' (Bynum 2006: 14). Cullen stated that it was analogous with magnetism or electricity (1781: 5).

The nocturnal wanderings of the somnambulist could also be seen as proof of the mechanical nature of moving without conscious volition. And, although the condition has been documented over the centuries by philosophers and physicians such as Plato, Aristotle, Galen and Hippocrates, to name a few, little has been discovered as to its cause. The condition, according to Colquhoun's introduction to Wienholt's work, has been attributed to either diabolical or divine agency, even into the nineteenth century (Colquhoun 1845: 10), so in order to shed some light on these antithetical positions it is necessary to give some explanation of the behaviours of somnambulists, and why they might be interpreted as automata. The relationship between natural somnambulism and 'artificial somnambulism' is highly pertinent, as is the latter's derivation from the practices of Viennese physician, Franz Anton Mesmer (1734–1815). Later in this chapter, Weinholt's focus on the peculiarity of somnambulists' sight, in the state of both natural and artificial somnambulism, will be illustrated with a few of the copious examples he documented, and Wienholt's own theory will be presented as to how somnambulists could see without perceptual vision.

This is intended as an overview of the subject of mesmerism and 'artificial somnambulism,' and cannot possibly cover the whole of this fascinating

---

2 For discussion of Luigi Galvani and Alessandro Volta's debate about animal electricity see Marco Bresadola's article: 'Animal Electricity at the End of the Eighteenth Century: The Many Facets of a Great Scientific Controversy' (2008).

topic. The main aim is to demonstrate how the shifts in human knowledge and the subsequent challenges to lived faith were overcome by thinkers in the early and mid-nineteenth century. The opportunity presented by the study of somnambulism, both artificial and natural, enabled some medical practitioners to try to establish proof of the transcendental within a medical-scientific framework.

SOMNAMBULISTS

Somnambulism translates as *sleep walking*, from the Latin words *somnus*, meaning sleep, and *ambulare*, meaning to walk about. There were two types of somnambulism: one natural, which occurred as part of a sleeping disorder, or other neurological condition; the second artificial, an induced somnambulistic state brought about via a practice such as 'animal magnetism.' The Marquis de Puységur, Amand Marie-Jacques de Chastenet (1751–1825), coined the condition 'magnetic sleep' (Tatar 1978: 27), and the effects produced by inducing this hypnotic state were proof, for some, of communion with the divine. Others sought to disparage the claims made by practitioners who induced 'magnetic sleep,' and others still, viewed the practice as diabolic. But it was the argument as to whether or not those in a trance state had use of their vision which was the definitive proof of the existence of the soul for physicians such as Arnold Wienholt, as will be examined later.

Somnambulism (both natural and artificial) was problematic for two main reasons. The first, according to reports, was that during the trance state the affected could not only undertake successfully those activities that they could do in a normal waking state, such as walking, talking or running, but also other activities that they could *not* do when awake. The second problem was that the affected, once awake, did not often remember their activities. Yet, when back in the somnambulistic trance, the sleeper seemed to pick up the track from the last time they were in the state. This indicated a double consciousness, which could be interpreted by some as indicating that human beings were machine-like beings, or automata without soul, or by others, that the sufferer was possessed. What sensory functions somnambulists had (in particular, sight) was a point of debate, and eminent physicians posited hypotheses about it, and conducted various experiments to test them. The most popular conclusion, drawn by many, was that the somnambulists were drawing upon their memory and imagination rather than actually using their sense of sight.

In Diderot and d'Alembert's *Encyclopédie* there is an extended entry on *Somnambulisme* in which the author, Ménuret de Chambaud, documented an incident related to him by the Archbishop of Bordeaux. The account describes the archbishop's encounter with a somnambulist whilst a young man at the seminary. According to the account, the somnambulist rose from his bed and sat at his desk composing sermons. What made this so remarkable, is that the young man did not appear to be using his eyes (de Chambaud 1765 Vol. 15: 341).[3] To test this, the observer placed a piece of card under the young man's chin, thereby obscuring the latter's view of his work. The young somnambulist continued to write and correct his work as if the card was not there, thereby confirming to the observer that he was not using his eyes (Vol. 15: 340-341). From this, de Chambaud concluded that 'some somnambulists have their eyes open, but it does not seem like they use them.'[4]

How those in trance states, such as somnambulism, could see without using their eyes caused much debate in the latter part of the eighteenth century, and at least the first half of the nineteenth century. Many eminent natural philosophers, such as the aforementioned William Cullen and also Erasmus Darwin (1731-1802), proffered highly influential definitions and explanations. The debate became entwined with investigations into a practice which Robert Darnton describes as a fad that became 'enmeshed with politics' in pre-revolutionary France (1976: 3). This practice was known as 'mesmerism,' named after the Viennese physician who developed it: Franz Anton Mesmer.

'ANIMAL MAGNETISM'

The treatment called 'mesmerism', referred to by Mesmer himself as 'animal magnetism' (Ellenberger 1981: 59), was a contentious issue in the late eighteenth century and at least until the middle of the nineteenth century, both in Britain and on the continent. Mesmerism became so popular that Louis XVI commissioned an inquiry to be conducted by eminent figures such as Benjamin Franklin and Antoine Lavoisier to investigate Mesmer's practices in Paris. They concluded that Mesmer's methods of obtaining

---

3 '*cette action faite sans le secours des yeux*'. My translation: this action is made without the eyes.
4 '*Quelques somnambules ont les yeux ouverts, mais il ne paroît pas qu'ils s'en servent*' (de Chambaud, 1765: Vol. 15, p. 341). '*Paroît*' here is taken to be *paraît* from *paraître*—to appear, seem. My translation.

cures for illnesses by way of inducing what he described as a 'magnetic crisis' in his patients, was little more than exploitation of imagination, and it was this that enabled cures (usually of nervous conditions) to be effected.

Mesmer's followers were undeterred by the findings of the inquiry and continued to practise and develop the methods. One such practitioner was the above-mentioned Marquis de Puységur, who, along with his brothers, discovered a condition brought about by 'animal magnetism' which induced what the Marquis described as a state of 'artificial somnambulism' (Ellenberger 1981: 71).

MESMER'S MAGNETIC PROCESS

Mesmer had theorised that there was an invisible, natural fluid that existed in and around humans and animals, and that this superfine fluid could be manipulated, via magnets, to effect cures for illness. Mesmer concluded that sickness occurred as a result of obstruction of the fluid, and that, by removing the obstruction and inducing what was described as a 'magnetic crisis,' the person would be cured (Darnton 1976: 6; Tatar 1978: 9, Ellenberger 1981: 59–60). Using magnets in a healing process was not a new idea, and Mesmer took the idea for his own treatments from Father Maximillian Hell, a Jesuit priest and professor of astronomy at the University of Vienna. Hell had been applying variously shaped steel magnets to the affected areas of his patients' bodies as a way to cure their ailments (Ellenberger 1981: 59, Fara 1995: 137, Tatar 1978: 9).

Mesmer filled bottles with iron filings and then arranged them in a formation like the spokes of a wheel in a covered tub (*baquet*) filled with magnetised water. Iron rods protruded and the patients would sit around the tub and apply the rods to the afflicted body part (Darnton 1976: 7–9, Ellenberger 1981: 64). A rope connected the patients to the *baquet* and to each other. Mesmer contributed to the atmosphere of his healing rooms through lavish décor and soothing music; he played the glass harmonica. According to one witness, the most 'sensible' effects were brought about by Mesmer himself, who would approach the patient and make certain movements with his eyes and hands.[5] Any patients who resisted the group process would be attended by Mesmer individually. He would sit the patient directly opposite to him, fixing the patient's knees between his own, and

---

5 '[T]he most sensible effects are produced on the approach of Mesmer, who is said to convey the fluid by certain motions of his hands or eyes, without touching the person' (John Grieve, quoted in Ellenberger 1981: 64).

then stare into the patient's eyes. Mesmer would then pass his hands over the patient's body 'searching for the obstacles impeding circulation of the magnetic fluid.' Then he would project the fluid 'emanating from his own eyes into those of the patient.' His active gaze was supposed not only to remove obstacles to the movement of the superfine fluid, but also immunise his patient against disease. Often these methods, the group and individual therapy, would send the patients into convulsions, described as a magnetic crisis, after which the curing of their ailments began to be discerned (Tatar 1978: 13–14).

The practice spread to the French colonies, specifically what later became Haiti—Saint Domingue.[6] 'Animal magnetism' was introduced to the slaves in Saint Domingue by Comte de Chastenet Antoine-Hyacinth de Puységur, brother to the Marquis, and the subsequent violence of the slaves was instrumental in the collapse of French dominion:

> In Saint-Domingue, magnetism degenerated into a psychic epidemic among the Negro slaves, increasing their agitation, and the French domination ended in a blood bath. Later Mesmer boasted that the new republic—now called Haiti—owed its independence to him. (Ellenberger 1981: 73)

Mesmer's method was extremely popular and other practitioners developed it, including the elder of the de Puységur brothers, Amand Marie-Jacques, Marquis de Puységur. It was this Puységur, neither physician nor scientist, whose discovery of 'artificial somnambulism' took the practice in a slightly different direction at the end of the eighteenth century in France.

'ARTIFICIAL SOMNAMBULISM'

Mesmer's practices initiated the setting up of Societies de l'Harmonie Universelle all over France which practised 'animal magnetism' with great success, until the French Revolution. The Marquis de Puységur and his brother joined the Parisian Society of Harmony when they were stationed in Paris. Once they retired from their military positions, they returned to the family home at Buzancy near Soissons, where they practised magnetism on the peasants working on their estate.

---

6 For an interesting discussion of the relationship between 'creole mesmerism' and psychoanalysis see Nathan Gorelick's article: 'Eximate Revolt: Mesmerism, Haiti, and the Origin of Psychoanalysis' (2013).

Puységur's practices led him to observe a particular type of trance state in his subject, Victor Race, a peasant who worked on the Puységurs' land. When in the magnetic trance, Victor was able converse on a more erudite level than was his usual level of communication. Puységur noticed that this type of trance rendered Victor into a state where he appeared to be awake. Also, during his magnetic trance Victor was able to articulate his innermost feelings, which he was unable to do when awake (Tatar 1978: 28; Ellenberger 1981: 45). In early 1785, Puységur travelled to Paris with Victor, demonstrating the trance condition. What Puységur hypothesised was that the condition and the cures were not brought about by the superfine fluid first theorised by Mesmer, but were instead effected by the practitioner's will (Ellenberger 1981: 72).[7]

Puységur, following Mesmer, had moved the practice from its supposed scientific roots to something else altogether. The lack of medical training required by practitioners, coupled with the cures seemingly effected by these very popular practices, were looked on with disfavour by physicians vying for business. To add to their displeasure, the non-medically trained Puységur, perhaps in a spirit of egalitarianism, had taught some of his patients to be practitioners.

THE SIGHTLESS SOMNAMBULISTS

Through Puységur's discovery, the similarity between somnambulism and 'animal magnetism' was firmly established. However, by the early nineteenth century, the practice of 'animal magnetism' had been debunked in France and ridiculed in British society. The phenomenon of the sightless somnambulists was explained, for the most part, as being the working of the imagination, in the same way that Benjamin Franklin, Antoine Lavoisier and the committee had debunked Mesmer's theories and explained his successes in 1794.

Similarly, the explanation that somnambulists' senses, such as vision, were excited by their imaginations was popular with many seeking to find a rational explanation for the successes of 'animal magnetism.' However, some such as Arnold Wienholt had a different hypothesis. Wienholt devoted much of the content of his seven lectures to presenting varying

---

7 Mesmer himself had begun to draw this conclusion when he realised that he could bring about a magnetic crisis simply by passing his hand over the subject, or even just looking at them.

respected opinions, from Erasmus Darwin for instance, and then systematically finding the flaws in their arguments. Wienholt's rebuttal of the popular theories adds weight to his own hypothesis that the sightlessness of somnambulists was indicative of a relationship with a divine power.

Darwin classified somnambulism as a disease of volition in his work *Zoonomia* (1794). The cause of it, he theorised, was the relief of pain through 'voluntary exertions' (Darwin 1794 Vol. I: 437). Darwin referred to it as a type of 'reverie,' which was very different to sleep. He stated that it arose from an excess of volition and argued that such conditions were of 'epileptic origin' and 'constituted another mode of mental exertion to relieve pain' (Vol. I: 437). This diagnosis of the condition indicates that there was a specific cause for the movements of somnambulists, rather than being automata. Darwin's view, based on others' accounts of somnambulists, was that the somnambulists were able to navigate their way around by opening their eyes briefly, but for the most part they used their imagination and so relied on their ideas of where things were positioned (Vol. I: 223-224). According to Wienholt, this erroneous (for him) hypothesis was prevalent in theories of somnambulism (Colquhoun 1845 [1805]: 58-59).

In Lecture II, Wienholt challenged this hypothesis: '[h]ow comes it that the perceptions and actions always correspond so exactly at the time, and with the external objects?' (Colquhoun 1845 [1805]: 56). Wienholt's argument was that, in a state of somnambulism, the eyes are not able to perceive; even if open, they are fixed and unresponsive (1845 [1805]: 78-79). Later, Wienholt made the point that those who were blind from birth could move about, and they could not be drawing upon memory and imagination as they would not have any prior experience, and thus no memory of visual perceptions. Wienholt described a blind lady whose blindness was not a hindrance to her selection of harmoniously coloured clothing; he argued that '[t]herefore there must be some other means of perception to supply the place of sight' (1845 [1805]: 123-5).

In order to illustrate his views, Wienholt drew upon many accounts of somnambulists not using their eyes. One case he considered to be very important in the construction of his argument was of a young somnambulist who uttered prayers and recited devotional sayings in the trance state. Then he would go outside and climb walls, and even climb up to a roof, sitting astride it and making as if he were riding a horse. On other occasions, he was able to use a needle and thread to mend clothes, all in the pitch dark. Having established that somnambulists' sightless vision is a recurring phenomenon, Wienholt spent much of the proceeding lectures presenting various theories, and detailing the nature of vision, specifically how the eyes are not able to function during the trance state, even if they are open.

DIVINE POWER OR DIABOLIC AGENCY?

By the time Colquhoun came to translate Wienholt's lectures in 1845, attitudes toward the trance states of natural and artificial somnambulism had changed, and many had begun to view it as having therapeutic potential, if not an indicator of the existence of the soul and its being empowered by the divine. There had been a revision of Mesmer's practices, and some practitioners had started to take these more seriously in terms of their medical application. That the somnambulist did not always recollect the somnambulistic wanderings once awake, but could pick them up again when in the state, was of interest and contributed to the formation of hypotheses about the unconscious mind. Puységur's development of 'artificial somnambulism' continued to be of interest, and throughout the nineteenth century developed into what James Braid called 'hypnotism' (Ellenberger 1981: 71). Similarly, the clairvoyant ability of some subjects was also acknowledged (Ellenberger 1981: 115).

Wienholt, in Lecture VI, had already drawn the conclusion that there must be another explanation for the blind being able to move freely, and somnambulists' ability to act without seeing. Wienholt described this as a 'sixth sense' and credited Puységur[8] with having stumbled across this idea some fifteen years prior to Wienholt's lecture (1845 [1805]: 125–126). Although the notion of a sixth sense was ridiculed, Wienholt described how it had gained traction when natural philosophers were trying to determine how bats could fly without sight. Earlier in his lectures, Wienholt described some unpleasant experiments on bats to determine that they were not using their eyes. The discovery that they used echolocation and sonar was over a century away.

To attribute this phenomenon of a sixth sense to humans was problematic since it was considered occult. In the introduction to Wienholt's lectures, Colquhoun described views held in the mid-nineteenth century:

The efficacy of animal magnetism...has been seriously alleged as depend[ing] on the co-operation of the devil, and the whole of the phenomena are

---

8 Ellenberger states that Mesmer had already described those with sensitivity to the magnetic fluid as having a sixth sense (1981: 78).

ascribed to diabolical agency, and it is a fact that these views have actually been inculcated and enforced from the pulpit. (Colquhoun 1845: xxii)

In a footnote, Colquhoun cited the Reverend George Sandby as reporting these attitudes in his 1848 work *Mesmerism and Its Opponents*. Sandby's own belief was that mesmerism was a blessing from God (Sandby 1848: vi), but this was not a view held by his contemporaries, such as the Reverend McNeile (Winter 1998: 260). Sandby described how his views made him the target of criticism: 'Superstition has its slaves in every spot; and I was soon pelted with pamphlets through the post, and made the mark for evil and ill-natured censure' (Sandby 1848: iv). Other critics of 'animal magnetism' practices included Mary Eddy Baker of the Christian Science movement, who warned her students of 'malicious animal magnetism,' describing it as 'evil thought' (Wilson 1961: 127). Mesmerism and 'artificial somnambulism' were regarded with suspicion not only as nefarious practices used by charlatans usurping the authority of the physician, but also, more sinisterly, as vehicles for the devil. This seeming regression to pre-Enlightenment thinking was perhaps not such a difficult leap to make. There is a tendency to assume that the rationalism of the Enlightenment completely displaced belief, but not only did its impact vary tremendously geographically, many people strove to incorporate their faith with rational approaches.

At the same time as Mesmer was enjoying success, a certain Father Gassner was conducting countless exorcisms across Swabia. Gassner, plagued by minor ailments, was convinced that his illness was caused by the devil, and when he performed an exorcism rite on himself, found relief. He set out to rid other devout folk of their ills via exorcism. This proved extremely efficacious, and in one summer alone he exorcised over three hundred nuns. The Munich Academy of Science, concerned about Gassner's discovery of so much apparent diabolic agency, sent Mesmer to investigate in 1775 (Ellenberger 1981: 60). Mesmer concluded that although the priest was a worthy and righteous man of God he was mistaken in the efficacy of exorcism, and Gassner was, without knowing it, a superb animal magnetist (Midelfort 2005: 65). In this instance, the secularity, and supposed science, of 'animal magnetism' was able to debunk faith. However, many men of science and faith claimed the practices of magnetism as a divine enterprise, and others, such as the Reverend McNeile, were convinced that it was a tool of the devil. There is some irony that Mesmer's own theories were debunked and ridiculed following the 1794 report, and then subsequently considered diabolic.

WIENHOLT'S THEORY OF SOMNAMBULIST'S SIGHT

There has not been room here to give full justice to the accounts of practitioners such as the Puységur brothers, but their experimentation with 'artificial somnambulism' as a mediumistic state for clairvoyance may be of interest and a fruitful line of enquiry might be found in the works referenced in this chapter. Similarly, those interested in pursuing the connection between magnetism and the diabolic will find Midelfort's work of interest, as well as that of the Reverend George Sandby, and also the rebuttal to the Reverend McNeile's criticism of Sandby by James Braid (1842). Ellenberger describes how the nature of magnetism was disputed, the arguments tending to be between those who adhered to a theory of magnetic fluid (the fluidists) and those who considered it to be a psychological phenomenon (the animists), as well as median paths (1981: 113). Throughout his lectures, Wienholt sought to create a logical path to his own theories about the somnambulist state and what it suggests about the immortality of the human soul. He enumerated various notable physicians' and philosophers' opinions and theories and systematically critiqued them. Early on he noted that the majority of the physiologists and psychologists whom he cited all opined that somnambulism was a median state between sleep and wakefulness (Colquhoun 1845 [1805]: 59).

Wienholt examined Erasmus Darwin's perspective in detail, criticising Darwin's lack of observed examples, and his interpretation of the young seminarian who Darwin suggested opened his eyes when he needed to see. Wienholt argued that de Chambaud's account suggested that this was not true. As has been outlined above, evidence for Wienholt's criticism can be found in de Chambaud's account. Wienholt's argument continued throughout his lectures with detailed comments on the condition of the eyes during the somnambulistic state. According to Wienholt, the eyes, particularly the iris, were immovable during somnambulism, and the pupil did not react to light (1845 [1805]: 78). Wienholt's contradiction of Darwin's hypothesis of somnambulism as being a form of reverie hinged on the point that, contrary to Darwin's view that the condition made senses insensible of external factors because the mind was preoccupied, some nerves of the skin or tongue appeared to be awake and able to transmit perceptions to the brain. Wienholt questioned why some senses should be capable of this while others are not. To further cement his argument against Darwin's hypothesis, Wienholt argued that given the physical immobility and non-reactive nature of the eyes, it would be very difficult for somnambulists to be able to use them to see (Colquhoun 1845 [1805]: 133–134).

Having established his arguments against these types of hypotheses, Wienholt presented his own in Lecture VII. He was very clear about the connection between natural and artificial somnambulism, and made the point that study of the natural state would shed light upon the artificial state. Interrogation of the conditions, Wienholt wrote, 'might lead to the contemplation of the objects of the supersensible world' (1845 [1805]: 130–131). What the investigations into somnambulism have proved, for Wienholt, is that this was evidence that the 'world within ourselves' is not restricted by the 'material laws of nature' and that immortality can be anticipated, even though the mortal body decays (1845 [1805]: 131).

What Wienholt argued is that in an altered state of consciousness, for example a somnambulistic trance, the body does not function in the same way as it does when awake, and so is not subject to the usual rules which govern the material body. And, if this is the case, he asked, 'how can we be certain about anything else' such as perception, and 'the laws which regulate the exercise of [...] mental powers?' (1845 [1805]: 131). Wienholt reasoned that in the trance state, the body's relationship with the soul is altered, and so the normal rules of the body's faculties do not apply. The dismissal of 'animal magnetism' as a quack practice, in Wienholt's view, had held back any real consideration of the supersensible world, and the relationship to a supersensible being, which he took as a given experience. Colquhoun added in a footnote that the practice of 'animal magnetism' had become popular again on the continent, and in Britain, but that it still went unacknowledged by 'many pretended learned men.' If serious study had been made of the phenomenon, then, Wienholt argued, the 'principle phenomena,' that is, of the vital principle, might have been found (1845 [1805]: 132–133).

Wienholt felt justified in stating that his investigations proved that the body could see without the use of the eyes:

> I am now entitled to hold it as demonstrated, that our soul, if it has once acquired perceptions through the medium of the eyes, may afterwards, in an incomprehensible manner, indeed, and without the use of this organ, receive similar impressions, and continue to remain in the same connection with the external world, in which it had previously stood by means of light and natural vision. (1845 [1805]: 136)

Here, Wienholt's use of *soul* appears to be the recipient of perceptual data, rather than being *perception* itself as contemporaries of Wienholt have sometimes meant.⁹

THE IMMORTAL SOUL

Wienholt outlined different faith positions in regard to the soul. The first was that some people believed that the thinking principle, the sense of self, would continue after death, and secondly some believed that the decayed body would reconstitute. Those without faith, he said, would find themselves uncertain in their opinion. The arguments he posed were that the spiritual powers depended on the body, and that external forces such as diet and climate affected the body. In this way he stated that the body and soul were inextricably linked (1845 [1805]: 137). The problem, as he saw it, was: How does anyone know what will happen after death? Is there a life eternal? What happens to the soul after the body has decayed?

Not content with throwing these metaphysical questions into his consideration of the nature of the soul, Wienholt argued that the soul needed the brain to create new impressions and ideas, and that without the physical body the eternal soul would never expand its ideas. Similarly, without the brain, how could the memory of self be preserved after death without the intervention of a miracle? The solution to these problems, he stated, was that the immateriality of the soul must be completely different from the body. Surely, he reasoned, if the somnambulist could see without the use of the eyes, then perhaps other organs could be substituted in the same way? Wienholt wrote:

> If an individual can acquire visual perceptions without the existence of the external organ, it is equally possible that, in another state, he may also be capable of thinking without the assistance of the brain, and that his imagination and memory may not be indissolubly attached to this soft and so easily destructible mass; that, on the contrary, the soul, in the exercise of its other functions, may as easily dispense with the latter, as vision may be manifested without the eyes. (1845 [1805]: 141)

To reinforce his ideas, he noted that somnambulists, once awake, do not remember the events of their somnambulistic state. This, Wienholt

---

9 As William Hughes warns in *That Devil's Trick* (2015), some references to soul made by various writers in the nineteenth century were using it as synonymous with perception.

stated, is evidence of the effect of a vital principle on the body and brain; he suggested that this principle or invisible power exerts a powerful influence on the mind when in sleep or a related condition. As outlined at the beginning of this chapter, Wienholt argued that the soul is bound up with the 'machine' of the human body, each influencing the other. But, the somnambulists provided for him evidence that in a trance they were unencumbered by their mortal bodies and selves, and so were free to be more perfect beings. The final proof for him was that the moral sensibilities of the somnambulists was heightened when in the state. This, for Wienholt, was proof that humans could develop spiritual faculties, so when a new body was conferred upon the spiritual self in the afterlife, it would be spiritually developed and ready for a perfected state.

Wienholt's arguments, very much a product of the rational, so-called Enlightenment period, demonstrate how hypotheses about the physical body, specifically here the use of sight without seeing, could be reasoned to incorporate not just a belief in the afterlife, but a perfected form of being human and a dynamic relationship with the invisible power of the divine. This integration of beliefs with those scientific discoveries demonstrated the tenacity of the belief in the divine nature of being human. Wienholt presented an insight into how this lived faith adapted and absorbed new perspectives, which it continues to do in the twenty-first century. And so, the sightlessness of the somnambulists, for Wienholt, was an indication of how, once unencumbered by that 'heavy external mantle [...] the spiritual I [...] will shine forth with a stronger and more brilliant lustre' (Colquhoun 1845 [1805]: 145–146).

REFERENCES

Braid, James. (1842) *Satanic Agency and Mesmerism Reviewed, in a Letter to the Reverend H. Mc.Neile, A.M. of Liverpool, in Reply to a Sermon Preached by Him in St. Jude's Church, Liverpool on Sunday April 10th, 1842*. Manchester: Simms and Dinham, Galt, and Anderson; Liverpool: Willmer and Smith.

Bresadola, Marco. (2008) 'Animal Electricity at the End of the Eighteenth Century: The Many Facets of a Great Scientific Controversy,' *Journal of the History of the Neurosciences*, 17(1), 8–32. https://doi.org/10.1080/09647040600764787

Bynum, W.F. (1994, 2006 edition) *Science and the Practice of Medicine in the Nineteenth Century*. New York: Cambridge University Press.

Colquhoun, J. C. (trans.) (1845). Wienholt, Arnold [1805], *Seven Lectures on Somnambulism*. Edinburgh: Adam and Charles Black; London: Longman, Green, Brown, and Longmans.

Cullen, William. (1781, second edition) *Lectures on the Materia Medica*. Dublin: W. and H. Whitestone.
Darnton, Robert. (1968, 1976 edition) *Mesmerism and the End of the Enlightenment*. Cambridge, MA: Harvard University Press.
Darwin, Erasmus. (1794) *Zoonomia*. London: J. Johnson.
De Chambaud, Menuret (eds. Denis Diderot and Jean d'Alembert). (1765) *Encyclopédie, ou, Dictionnaire raisonné des sciences, des arts et des métiers*, Tome Quinzième. France: A. Neufchastel, Chez Samuel Faulche et Compagnie, et Libraires, Imprimeurs.
Ellenberger, Henri. (1981, 1970) *The Discovery of the Unconscious: The History and Evolution of Dynamic Psychiatry*. New York: Basic Books.
Fara, Patricia. (1995) 'An Attractive Therapy: Animal Magnetism in Eighteenth-Century England,' *History of Science*, XXXIII(2), 127–177. https://doi.org/10.1177/007327539503300201
Gorelick, Nathan. (2013) 'Eximate Revolt: Mesmerism, Haiti, and the Origin of Psychoanalysis,' *CR: The New Centennial Review*, 13(3), 115–138. https://doi.org/10.1353/ncr.2013.0027
Hughes, William. (2015) *That Devil's Trick: Hypnotism and the Victorian Popular Imagination*. Manchester: Manchester University Press.
Midelfort, Eric. (2005) *Exorcism and Enlightenment: Johann Joseph Gassner and the Demons of Eighteenth-Century Germany*. New Haven, CT: Yale University Press.
Sandby, George. (1848, second edition) *Mesmerism and Its Opponents*. London: Longman, Brown, Green, and Longmans.
Tatar, Maria. (1978) *Spellbound: Studies on Mesmerism and Literature*. Princeton, NJ: Princeton University Press.
Thomas, Keith. (1991, 1971) *Religion and the Decline of Magic*. St Ives, UK: Penguin.
Wilson, Bryan, R. (1961) *Sects and Society: A Sociological Study of the Elim Tabernacle, Christian Science, and the Christadelphians*. Berkeley: University of California Press.
Winter, Alison. (1998) *Mesmerized: Powers of Mind in Victorian Britain*. Chicago: University of Chicago Press.

Martina Bartlett is currently reading for a PhD at Winchester University in the UK. The focus of her thesis is on the work of John William Polidori, who was physician to Lord Byron, as well as being a poet and author in his own right. Polidori's most notable work was *The Vampyre* (1819), and Martina is examining this, and his other literary works, in light of his medical thesis on somnambulism. She is a member of The Folklore Society, and gave a paper at their 'Reflected Shadows: Folklore and the Gothic' conference in 2016. She is also a member of The Romanticism Association, and delivered a paper at their inaugural conference 'Supernatural Romanticism' in Strasbourg, 2017. Martina also delivered a paper on Polidori's novel *Ernestus Berchtold, or The Modern Oedipus* at the 'Frankenstein Unbound' conference in 2018.

Chapter 7

The Experience of Seeing: Spirit Possession as Performance

BETTINA E. SCHMIDT

Sight is probably one of the most difficult senses for an anthropologist to deal with, but one of the most fascinating as well. Seeing involves the subjective perspective of the anthropologist who also has to remain objective. Participant observation that is based on the experience of the Other is still the hallmark of anthropology. During ethnographic research all of our senses are involved and we reflect on what we hear, see and even touch, smell and taste. But how can we interpret objectively what we gather via our subjective senses? For some, chaos might be an expression of life and for others chaos might be experienced negatively. Some connect dark colours with feelings of despair while others cherish them. Sight is one of the key senses for any ethnographic research but also very difficult to rely on. In the past anthropologists have therefore often ignored their own perception of what they saw, and in their publications they have focused on numbers, measurements and other so-called scientific features. However, anthropology has moved on and acknowledges now the impact of our own experience during fieldwork. Nevertheless, we still have some way ahead of us.

In this chapter I will discuss my experience of seeing spirit manifestations within Caribbean and Brazilian religions with African roots, my main research area. These manifestations take place usually during community rituals and are perceived as cherished occasions as the divine spirits are regarded as having positive influence on human beings. At the core of it is the concept of *ashe* (also written *axe* in Brazil or *ache* in Cuba), a spiritual force or energy that is in all living beings (see Schmidt 2012). Without *ashe* there would be no life. *Ashe* is given by the divine creator and is perceived as fluid. Some actions can cause *ashe* to diminish, while other actions can increase *ashe*. Interaction with divine spirits, the *orishas* (also written *orixas* or *orichas*) is perceived as positive as it increases *ashe*. Hence, when the *orishas* manifest themselves during ceremonies, the community is blessed and *ashe* grows in the participating individuals.

This is (in short) the theological explanation of why spirit manifestations are perceived as positive for all living beings. However, British anthropologists are usually more interested in the practice and less in theological explanation. As we have already learnt from E. E. Evans-Pritchard, religion is what people do and not what they say they believe in. When we focus on the practice of spirit manifestation, sight gains significance and therefore also our experience of seeing. Hence, analysing what we see and how we understand what we see is the key way of engagement for an anthropologist of religion. I have chosen some of my own experiences with seeing spirit manifestations as the basis for discussing the problems with the experience of seeing. The spirit manifestations were, of course, not performed for me, hence I was never the intended audience. But, as I will show in this chapter, my experience of seeing and my emotional reaction to what I saw provide a bridge to understanding the point of view of the devotees. My argument is therefore that sight allows researchers to incorporate the experience of seeing into the analysis of a ritual.

The chapter is divided in two parts and in each of these I will refer to excerpts from my field diary as an illustration of the problem around seeing. In the first section I have included an excerpt from my New York field diary which describes one of the first spirit manifestations I was able to observe. I will use my experience to discuss the limitations of analysing what we see, and highlight some of the key problems that are linked to an ethnocentric and very narrow definition of performance. In the second part I will reflect on a more recent experience with spirit manifestation in São Paulo. I will use two short observations from my field diary to acknowledge the importance of the experience of seeing for anthropologists. Hence, the overall focus of this chapter is on the *experience* of seeing. While we teach our students the features of participant observation, we often overlook reflecting on our own experience during fieldwork. Can we rely on what we see? How can we reflect on what we see when we are not sure of its 'authenticity'? And how do we bring in the participants' point of view? I will argue that if we reflect more on the *experience* of seeing and less on the virtues of participant *observation* we can start a dialogue between our experience of seeing and the emic experience of practising.

THE OVERWHELMING POWER OF SEEING: THE PERFORMANCE OF SPIRIT MANIFESTATIONS

Though I had studied religions with spirit manifestations for my PhD, which focused on two vernacular traditions in Puerto Rico, it was not until I began my research on Caribbean religions in New York City some years later that I was allowed to attend ceremonies with spirit manifestations. During my previous study in Puerto Rico I had some encounters with spirits within Puerto Rican spiritism but I was not invited to attend Santeria ceremonies with elaborate spirit manifestations. I was told that they would be too dangerous for me as an outsider as I would not be able to handle the manifestation of a spirit if one approached me. As my PhD was on identity and religion, I was able to undertake my research without observing any ceremonies with spirit manifestations by speaking with several priests, priestesses and ordinary members of various communities. But I knew something was missing.

In New York, during my research on the Caribbean Diaspora, I was able to attend several ceremonies, usually due to introductions by musicians who became some of my gate-keepers in this project. My research at that time focused on three Caribbean religions, Vodou from Haiti, Shango from Trinidad and Tobago, and Santeria from Cuba. While my research was on questions concerning Diaspora communities in the light of cultural theory and not on religious practices, the memories of attending these ceremonies impacted on my experience with the Caribbean Diaspora and influenced my later research on spirit possession and trance. Here is an excerpt from my notes on one of the first ceremonies I attended. It was a very cold day and I had been invited to attend a ceremony in the Yoruba-Orisha Baptist Church in Brooklyn by the Reverend of the Church whom I had interviewed previously. As I was told it was the celebration of the anniversary of the Church, I was unprepared for the manifestation that happened during the ceremony (**Figure 7.1**).

The blaze of colour was overwhelming. The whole church building was painted and decorated in honour of the 23rd anniversary of its foundation. In the background was the altar on a podium, with chairs for the most important members and the guest of honour. In front the benches for the singers and the children were lined up. I was fascinated in particular by the Stations of the Cross: side by side with Christian saints I noticed a figure of Buddha and of a Native American, important religious symbols in the pantheon of the Yoruba-Orisha Baptist Church. The congregation represented itself as a place for many religions.

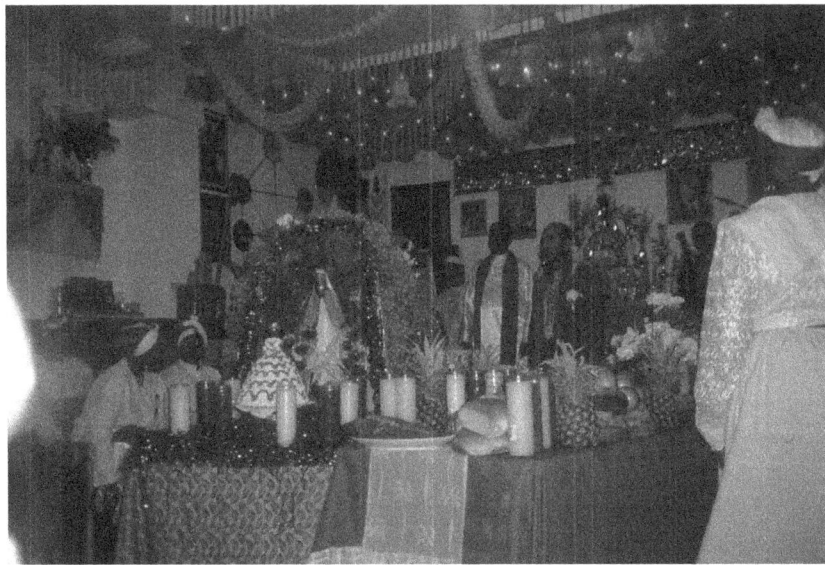

Figure 7.1 Ceremony in the Yoruba-Orisha Baptist Church in Brooklyn, New York City. Photo by Bettina E. Schmidt, 15 February 1998.

The celebration started only slowly. One by one the members arrived. The women and girls were dressed in brilliant white and blue dresses with matching scarves, the men in suits. On one side of the hall were two tables with food; and in front of the altar a small table with a grotto made out of grapes that contained the statue of the Virgin of Lourdes, the patron of the congregation. After an hour some women began to hum religious hymns. Finally one woman started the singing, soon joined by other women. A man began to drum and the service started.

There was an impressive mood in the hall. The air became more and more muggy; the women, who had noticed and greeted every newcomer in the beginning, changed the hall into a sacred place with their voices. Their singing and the drum music seemed to rise to the sky or at least to the Caribbean, away from the cold and wet atmosphere of Brooklyn. Every time the music started to slow down, the minister or one of his assistants tried to push the women to sing louder. As I was told later, only music can create a successful service because the power of the music can call the Holy Spirit to Earth.

The first part of the service contained the last part of a novena, a series of services. Two mothers in the congregation led the recitation of the rosary. There was repeated singing, followed by speeches, the welcoming of the guests and lectures from the Bible. Singing and drumming became louder and louder. Some members started to feel the presence of the Holy Spirit. They twitched and shrugged. When someone began to behave wildly, members of the congregation immediately attended to them so that they did not injure themselves or others.

During a break the secretary read some letters to the congregation; more speeches were given, members were honoured with awards, and the children of the Sunday school sang some songs. Then the tables with the food were put in the central part of the hall. The second part began. The (male) minister had changed into a white and blue dress with a scarf. The room was nearly airless. The music was booming in our ears. The manifestation of the Holy Spirit intensified. Around me more and more women fell into trance. Some of them could barely stand despite the support of their attendants. They fell to the floor, pushed against each other and pressed others against the wall. It was totally chaotic. Even the assistants seemed to have lost the overview. The music became more and more powerful. Finally the minister fell into trance. In this state he anointed the congregation with his oily hands until he fell to the floor unconscious and had to be carried away to his flat above the hall.

Then a woman was possessed by Saint Michael, i.e. Ogun. Someone gave her a lance, and she whirled through the hall despite the crowd of people standing in it. Even in trance she seemed to know what to do. At least this was what I hoped when she approached me. The assistants of the minister tried to end the service but the women ignored them. The two factions started to argue about who was in charge of the event when the minister returned and took control again. Slowly the crowd became quieter. After another hour the service came to an end and the shared dinner started. (Previously published in Schmidt 2008: 87–89)

As the excerpt shows, I was overwhelmed by the experience. The church was colourfully decorated, church members in their Sunday clothing and the church elders (women and men) nicely dressed. Together with the drums and singing, the candles and the smell, I felt fully engaged with all my senses. But what to do with such an experience? I used the excerpt previously as an illustration of the ritual practice of the community. However, the research aim was linked to an understanding of cultural bricolage and my analysis focused on cultural theories. I struggled with finding an appropriate method which would allow me to include my experience of these ceremonies into the wider theoretical discussion.

The interpretation of practices in the realm of religious or spiritual traditions is probably the most difficult within anthropology. While participation in rituals is fascinating, as my excerpt has shown, to make sense of what we see is extremely difficult. I began by looking at Performance Studies as a way out of my problem. Performance Studies has helped anthropologists to appreciate the performative skills of the participants. As Mark Münzel states: 'While I cannot accept explanation given by millions of Brazilian believers that the divinity Xango is really present, I do not want to denigrate their experience either by reducing it to psycho-social or other factors in arrogant presumptuousness. I prefer to say that I do not understand what is going on. But I am searching for a level at which I can share some common feeling with these Brazilian believers: one small area would be the admiration for the great spectacle' (Münzel 1994: 143). We can acknowledge the work participants have invested in manufacturing the costumes and decorations, the skills of the musicians and dancers, and the overall choreography of the performance.

However, when I tried to analyse Caribbean ceremonies using the Performance Studies approach (Schmidt 2002, 2008), I realised its limitation derived from its ethnocentric concept of theatre, which was at the core of Performance Studies at that time. While the collaboration of Performance Studies scholars such as Richard Schechner and Eugenio Barba with anthropologists such as Victor Turner opened the way for understanding other cultures and their theatrical performances, they also limited our understanding due to the restricted nature of the European definition of 'theatre' (Mandressi 1996: 91–93). I also realised that the emic perspective of the participants was put aside as the focus was on the theatrical performance. The French School of *ethnoscénologie* offers an alternative that allows us to maintain academic scrutiny and appreciate the emic perspective without pre-judging it from a Western perspective. Instead of limiting the focus to theatrical performances, scholars from this school study all kinds of body movements, whether they are connected to theatre, ritual or dance. Jean-Marie Pradier, one of the founding scholars of the school, defines *spectaculaire* (performing) as:

> 1) that one should not reduce it only to visual items; 2) that it does not only refer to ensembles of modalities of human perspective; 3) that it embraces all different human manifestations, including somatic, physical, cognitive, emotional, and spiritual dimensions [1) *ne se réduit pas au visuel; 2) se réfère à l'ensemble des modalités perceptives humanes; 3) souligne l'aspect global des manifestations émergentes humaines, incluant les dimensions somatiques, physiques, cognitives, émotionnelles et spirituelles*]. (Pradier 1996: 17, my translation)

Consequently, all kinds of body movements are included under this umbrella and can be studied in the same way, whether they are dance movements or rituals, art or street dance, shamanism or other ceremonies and even music (Pradier 1996: 37). Following this approach, I decided to include in my study of Caribbean communities in New York City not only observations of rituals but also theatrical performances, dance workshops, exhibitions, parades and the Caribbean Carnival (**Figure 7.2**). Performance Studies include, of course, also studies of several of these activities. However, *ethnoscénologie* distances its research from the European idea of entertainment and considers the emic perspective. Armindo Bião, for instance, harshly criticises scholars who regard Brazilian forms of spirit possession rituals as inferior to African ones due to the syncretic nature of Afro-Brazilian religions (Bião 1996: 149–151). One of these scholars is Gilbert Rouget, who differentiates between different degrees of trance and describes spirit manifestation in Candomblé as minor in comparison to the Yoruba spirit manifestations in Nigeria, Benin and Togo (Rouget 1996: 52–53). Bião, on the other hand, argues against the ethnocentrism by European intellectuals and insists on the significance of Candomblé and its form of trance as the central cultural element in Salvador da Bahia (Bião 1996: 149–151). Stepping along his footpath, I argue that the assessment of a spirit manifestation with regard to authenticity is irrelevant because this distinction is to be made only by the participants and not by the scholar

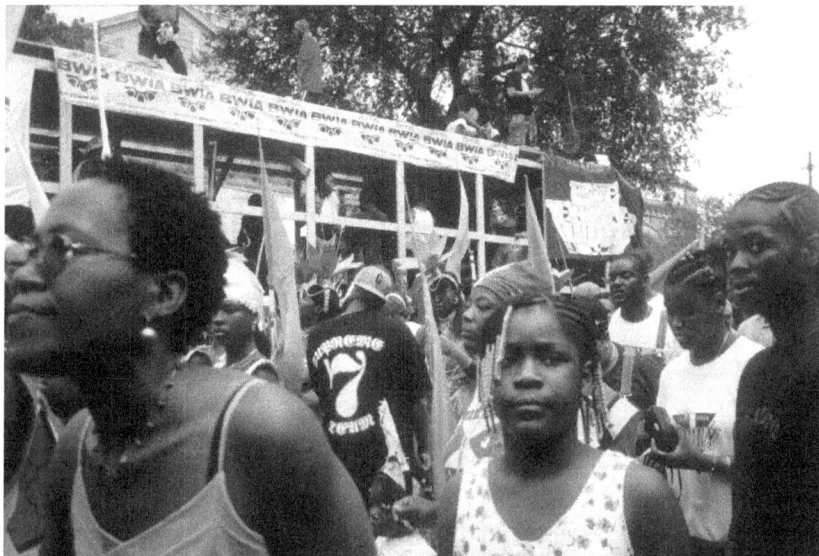

Figure 7.2 Caribbean Carnival parade in Brooklyn, New York City. Photo by Bettina E. Schmidt, 6 September 1999.

(see also Schmidt 2016). We can learn from the reaction of the participants whether they accept the presence of a spirit (and its identity), as the following memory demonstrates.

During my research of the Caribbean Diaspora in New York I attended once a theatrical performance of traditional Haitian dances, which included in the second part of the performance some so-called Vodou dances. While there were many Haitian immigrants among the audience, it was clearly aimed to entertain a wide audience without specific knowledge of the culture and the religion. Baron Samdi and other popular and recognisable spiritual entities formed part of the performance. It was clearly staged, though I recognised among the musicians and dancers several people from Vodou ceremonies. Even the *mambo*, the priestess of one of the Vodou temples I had visited and interviewed for my research, was one of the dancers. However, the main dancer was a young woman I had also seen previously at a Vodou ceremony, though only at the periphery, as a visitor.

Suddenly the atmosphere on stage changed and I noticed that a man who was sitting in the front row and whom I recognised as the assistant of the *mambo* got nervous. Then he stood up and walked from the side entrance onto the stage straight to the musicians. Sharply he gave the master drummer who was in charge of the performance an instruction and immediately the music changed. What had happened? Performances on stage are regarded as entertainment and secular events. A spirit should not manifest though the manifestation is played out. However, the musicians (who also played regularly at Vodou ceremonies) were very good and had—unintentionally—attracted a Vodou spirit who began to approach the *mambo*. Her movements had changed as her body experienced the approach of one of her Vodou spirits. Her assistant saw the change in her body movements and realised at once what was going on. In an effort to prevent a full spirit manifestation, he ordered the musicians to change the rhythm so that the spirit would no longer be attracted.

This small episode had helped me to understand some of the internal structures of the Caribbean Diaspora communities in New York. But for the purpose of this chapter the scene highlights the importance of precise observation of human behaviour. Instead of describing in detail the dance movements and the costumes, I reflected on behaviour, and in particular on non-ordinary behaviour, as a way in which we can learn to assess spirit manifestation from an emic perspective. The issue here was not whether the body movements were well performed but whether it was proper to initiate embodiment of a spirit while on stage. Hence, non-verbal information such as body language can inform us about a hidden agenda, sometimes even about something people would hesitate to express in words but consciously and deliberately express through body language. The problem with such information is the difficulty to record. As I reflected earlier, 'we cannot quote information based on an attitude expressed through body language in the same way as we can quote information given in an interview. Nevertheless body language can carry important information that is otherwise difficult to get. It is possible to hide one's opinion in an interview but often impossible in body language' (Schmidt 2008: 21).

This is particularly the case in research on religions. Already, my PhD research in Puerto Rico had showed me how difficult it is to study phenomena such as trance and spirit possession that often are at the periphery of mainstream religious practices. The result is that we have problems interpreting them. How can I analyse something I do not experience and sometimes cannot even observe? I can, of course, describe the performance. But I cannot tell whether the spirit is speaking or the human body. However, as I learnt from *ethnoscénologie*, 'understanding implies a process of creative and inter-subjective observation.... Instead of struggling with my fascination for Caribbean religions, I allowed them to overwhelm me' (Schmidt 2008: 22).

The experience of being overwhelmed reflects a notion that the German anthropologist Adolf Ellegard Jensen described as *Ergriffenheit*. Jensen presented *Ergriffenheit* as the key to new academic knowledge: One has to become overwhelmed (*ergriffen*) to create something new, including academic understanding (Jensen 1992: 23). While sometimes wrongly translated as 'emotion' or 'inspiration,' *Ergriffenheit* is more. Jensen was part of the Frankfurt school of cultural morphology founded by Leo Frobenius. Nowadays often overlooked or criticised due to—as Gingrich writes—the 'school's overt preference for the irrational and the aesthetic' (2005: 108), Jensen's form of cultural morphology has some similarities, as Gingrich outlines, to the work of Ruth Benedict in the Boas tradition of the USA as well as to Marcel Griaule's school. Common in these three strands is the ethnographical richness of their work, though for many, including Gingrich, Jensen's impact 'remained a mysticist and particularist theoretical influence' (2005: 140). This critique echoes other criticism against scholars working on religious or spiritual experiences. Instead of remaining on the outside, Jensen tried to express in his concept of *Ergriffenheit* a different way of learning that allows a wider engagement with our experience of seeing, even though he was not really concerned with the sense but with ideas.

While the term *Ergriffenheit* therefore does not really describe the act of seeing, I view it as connected to the experience of seeing nonetheless. It highlights that seeing is just the first—though significant—step to understanding. The crucial feature is that our experience of seeing—embedded in a dialogue with practitioners about their understanding of what has happened—becomes the starting point of the interpretation of religious and spiritual practices. This also means that one does not need to become an insider to become *ergriffen* by an experience. It is also possible to share some of the notion of the experience without embodying the spirit.

I still have not analysed the ceremony in detail but used it to demonstrate my approach. I do not share their experience, nor is my cultural, religious or even ethnic background similar to theirs. Growing up within the German Lutheran Church which cherishes hymns and prayers but not the embodiment of the divine, I have little in common with the members of the Yoruba-Orisha Baptist Church in New York City. But the emotion of *Ergriffenheit* during their anniversary of the church in Brooklyn created a bridge between our worlds and allowed me a glimpse into their experience.

CAN WE RELY ON OUR SIGHT? THE SUBJECTIVITY OF SEEING EMBODIED SPIRITS

The debate about how to deal with the overwhelming impression of spirit manifestations is just one aspect of the debate about the experience of seeing. Another one is about the subjectivity of the experience itself. Despite the post-colonial turn to embrace the position of the Other, we have seen an increasing debate about the significance of experience, in particular among scholars in the study of religions. In an effort to distinguish their field of study from theological positions, religious studies scholars have a problem with experience. It is problematic for many even to acknowledge the value of experience as it would seem to valorise 'experience' above 'scientific verification,' the 'subjective' over the 'objective' (Sharf 1998; see also McCutcheon 2012). Sharf's famous example refers to reports of alien abduction: While there is common agreement that alien abductions never happened, there are many personal reports about them which should, according to Sharf, be read as religious narratives like any other reports of experiences by mystics or shamans (Sharf 1998: 110). In the end it depends on the understanding of people having the experience and not on the verification of the experience. However, for others this argument is too far-reaching and interferes with academic standards.

At this point I shall present another excerpt from my field diary, this time from my research about spirit possession and trance in Brazil. Spirit possession has fascinated me for a long time, although I avoided it in my previous projects on the study of the core practice. First, I focused on issues of identity without touching the emic understanding of the practice apart from acknowledging it. Later, when studying Caribbean religious communities in New York City, I had the occasion of attending several rituals in different communities and had at last first-hand experience with the practice usually labelled spirit possession, though strictly as a distant observer. And my post-doctoral thesis focused on cultural theory and Diaspora. Years later, when I moved from anthropology to the study of religions, I decided to develop a new project, focusing this time on the understanding of spirit possession and trance. As a research location I choose Brazil, which has a range of traditions with different forms of mediumship practice. During my research I interviewed priests, priestesses and ordinary members of various communities of Candomblé, Umbanda and other Afro-Brazilian traditions as well as different forms of spiritism and Charismatic Christianity, and attended

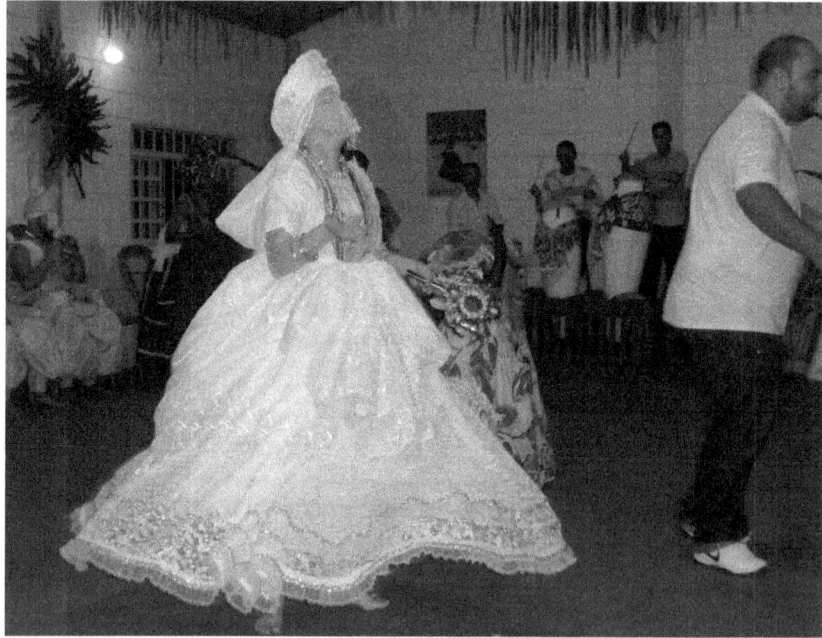

Figure 7.3 Candomblé ceremony in São Paulo. Photo by Bettina E. Schmidt, 24 April 2010.

ceremonies with spirit manifestations in different communities of these traditions. I became fascinated in particular by the colourful ceremonies of the Candomblé tradition (**Figure 7.3**). However, for the purpose of this article I will reflect on two occasions from other traditions, Umbanda and Spiritism, that are less colourful. The common link between these two observations is body size, or, more precisely, how my eye saw the body shapes of the same people differently, depending on whether I saw them during a ceremony, in the moment of spirit manifestation, or in the outside world, while conducting an interview.

On 19 March 2010, I attended an Umbanda ceremony for the spiritual entities called preto velho in Campinas, São Paulo State. I was given a lift from São Paulo by two filhas de santo, young women, initiated members of the Umbanda community I was about to visit. My transport was arranged by the mãe de santo, the priestess and founder of this community, whom I had met already a few times in São Paulo. Our first meeting had taken place on the University campus and I had been impressed by her presence. Afterwards I arranged to interview her and during this interview she invited me to attend a ceremony in her terreiro. The two young women talked during our car journey mainly about common friends and social activities and I could hardly get a question about their beliefs and practices into the conversation.

Upon arrival they introduced me to the other members of the community and showed me around. The priestess was already getting ready for the ceremony and unable to see me. I was then asked to sit down and wait with other clients in a dedicated area, just outside of the sacred circle. Some more people arrived though overall the audience that night remained small. Once in a while, other members arrived and walked to the back of the terreiro and I could hear some conversations and singing. While I waited for the ceremony to begin, I noticed small stools and very short walking sticks, situated around the room. The priestess was a very tall woman, as were most of the other members I had met, so I had no idea for whom they were set up. They looked like stools for children and usually no children attended these ceremonies, in particular not in the centre of the ritual space.

The evening went as other ceremonies I attended. The drums were brought in, the musicians started, people began to sing and then the mediums walked slowly into the central space, accompanied by assistants. After a while the audience was allowed to approach the mediums in order to present their problems and questions. As in other ceremonies, I also approached the mediums and consulted the spirits. And suddenly I realized that the stools no longer looked too small. Even the small sticks next to them looked the right size for walking canes for the mediums.

The ceremony on that day was for the preto velho entities that represent spirits of the old Black Brazilians. The mediums resembled very old, bent people who could hardly walk and needed to lean on the walking canes. The size of the stools that made no sense to me before the ceremony was perfectly fine as soon as the mediums incorporating the preto velho walked in.

Something similar had happened in a Spiritist centre. I visited the centre for the first time on 30 March 2010 and was able to observe a healing session (cura espiritual). When I came back a few weeks later in order to observe another different healing session (terapêutica spiritual), this time a so-called desobsessão, I had arranged to interview the woman who had worked as the main medium during my earlier visit. Hence, in this case I met her first as a medium incorporating a spirit of a healer before seeing her again in her secular self and conducting an interview. Standing next to her I suddenly realised that she was shorter than me. When I observed her during my earlier visit, treating patients while incorporating her spirit guide, I had thought that she was quite a tall person, definitely taller than me. But in her 'normal' state I realised that my perception was wrong.

This short reflection on my own experience of seeing bodies of mediums changed due to the incarnation of spirits addresses the important issue of how much we can rely on what we see. I did not measure any of the mediums and have therefore no means to scientifically prove what I saw. And, to be honest, I am not interested in measurements but in the body as a whole as well as the perception of the body. My research aim was not to determine whether it may have been a psychological or physiological phenomenon but how it was interpreted by those to whom it happened. During my interviews, I asked the mediums therefore how the experience affected them, emotionally or physically. One interviewee, a woman trained as a medium in a Kardecist centre (though she did not work as a medium at the time of the interviews), said when I asked her how the first experience felt:

> I do not remember anything about the first time except that the sensation was a strong heat, the sensation of heat and sleep at the same time. I felt a huge weight in my back and neck, and I began to feel my heart. The heart accelerated! And it was the sensation of two hearts beating inside me. There was a kind of force in my throat, a very strong energy in the throat, and I felt like it was about to speak.

And she continued later:

I felt the voice leaving my body, but unlike other people who do not have consciousness, I found that only a fraction of me was not conscious.... I felt that the person spoke in my head, I heard [the voice] and spoke [at the same time]. At times I was afraid of not speaking correctly, or that the person speaking was me [and not the spirit]. As it passed I thought, 'ah, was it only in my imagination?' ... But as time passed, I had ideas that I never had before. And this was the biggest sensation. I felt an embrace. I had no more doubts. (Interview on 27 May 2010)

She furnished, in this interview and in later conversations, a very graphical description of the physical impact the spirit manifestation had on her. Most interviewees highlighted the feeling of a form of energy when I asked them to describe how the encounter felt, and often explained that the energy differs depending on the spiritual entity. One interviewee, a priestess who is initiated in Umbanda and Candomblé, tried to explain to me how it felt using the analogy of anaesthesia:

It's different, the *orixá* [Candomblé] has a stronger vibration than an entity [in Umbanda]. It's a vibration; it is something that takes you, which has force. But the sense is different in Umbanda. There are various kinds of spirit, in the same way that people are also different. In my experience—have you ever had surgery? And were given an injection of a drug, an anaesthetic before the surgery? You stay well and then you do not remember anything more because the anaesthesia puts you to sleep? The state is not the same, but it is very similar. (Interview on 16 March 2010)

But perhaps the best example is this excerpt from an interview with an Umbanda priest who discusses the impact of alcohol on the body of the human medium. Within Umbanda ceremonies, the spirits like to party, hence they frequently ask for alcohol during the spirit manifestation (**Figure 7.4**). I discussed with the priest the differences of the spirit manifestations and he tried to explain the lack of control while remaining conscious at the same time with alcohol:

In the case of Umbanda it varies from entity to entity.... In one case I have full awareness of what is happening. In other cases I have full consciousness, but I cannot control the movements. There are also others where I can master the moves, but I cannot control the voice. There are some who do not speak, but have a special way to hinder me, one entity, for instance, with drinking. The taste of alcohol leaves me unconscious because of the alcohol. However, [during the incorporation] I am aware of his attitude when he is drunk, but when he leaves, I do not have the characteristics of being drunk.

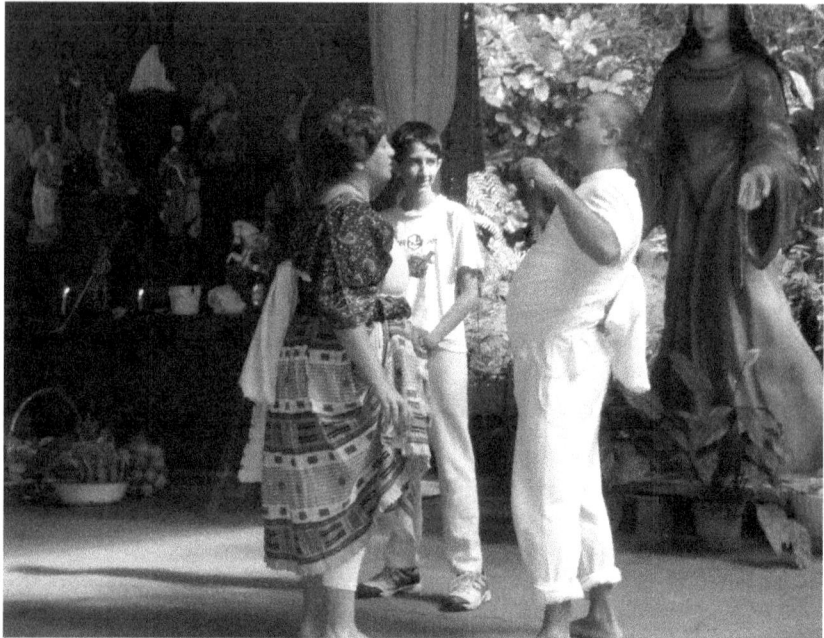

Figure 7.4 Umbanda ceremony in São Paulo. Photo by Bettina E. Schmidt, 11 April 2010.

In this case, if I could check the percentage of alcohol in my blood, there would certainly be alcohol there. But I do not have the same feeling when I'm drunk. This is because I did not [remember] that I drank so badly. I have no visual distortions, [but] there is a specific entity that does that! It does not allow me to know what the entity is saying. As if he [the spiritual entity] realizes that I'm conscious, and makes me, one way or another, unconscious! If I do not get unconscious for good, another less pleasant way is by alcohol. (Interview on 14 April 2010)

While he normally does not like alcohol and does not drink, during the spirit manifestation the spirit is in control and he drinks but afterwards he claims to be not drunk.

These excerpts from some of my interviews support my own impression that spirit manifestation can transform the body of the human mediums (see also Schmidt 2014). But these are, of course, not scientific evidence. As the last interviewee said, he did not measure the amount of alcohol in his blood during and after the spirit manifestation. What he presented were merely subjective impressions. The same is true for my own experiences—

I did not measure anyone but recall in the excerpts from my field diary just my own impressions of different body shapes.

Hence, what I present here are not physical facts but subjective impressions. And as Peter Fenwick (2001) points out, it is difficult, probably impossible, to scientifically evaluate and explain subjective experience. But I argue that these subjective recollections enable us to gain insight into spirit manifestations. Johannes Fabian (2002) has argued that knowledge is not 'an object that can be objectively observed rather than a process' and knowledge 'depends on actual, embodied people in real historical time, sharing a physical and social space, engaging in linguistic and practical performances and exchanges' (summarised by Bowie 2012: 1). The experience of seeing spirit manifestation even as an observer can lead to new knowledge due to the shared physical space and, as I argued in the first section of this chapter, becomes the bridge between our experience of seeing and their embodied experience of the spirit manifestation. Fiona Bowie even argues that we need to develop a new methodology, which she describes as empathic engagement, because 'mind, emotions and body are all involved in the production of anthropological knowledge' (2012: 1). She further explains that 'Empathy and engagement imply that there is no point embarking on a study with a set of fixed ideas or outcomes. One needs to be open to the experience and willing to learn with one's body (senses) and emotions, as well as one's intellect' (Bowie 2012: 2).

Bowie follows here in the footsteps of Edith Turner (1992, 1993) who is one of the pioneers of anthropology of experience. Bowie describes it as 'alternative anthropological tradition' which is based on an 'experiential lineage' (2016: 21). However, while the inclusion of one's own experience is quite common in studies of initiatory religions such as the Afro-American religions, the step to become initiated only in order to gain knowledge that is usually restricted to initiated devotees is controversial. Knowledge gained through initiation is considered sacred and limited to people who have passed the initiation (see Evans-Pritchard's problem in getting information about the Azande 'witchcraft' training [1976]).

Where does this leave me in light of a better understanding of spirit manifestation? I am no step further in recognising whether a spirit of a doctor of medicine treats the patients in a Spiritist centre; whether an *orixá* conveys his or her pleasure about the presence of so many clients; or whether a *caboclo* criticises me for an incorrect movement. I do not understand how a woman with a disfigured foot can dance for hours without pain; why a man wakes up from his trance feeling immensely sad about the loss of his *orixá*; or why someone who has consumed an enormous amount of alcohol exhibits no effects. Pyysiäinen defines religion as 'a concept that identifies the personalistic counter-intuitive representations and the related practices, institutions, etc. that are widely spread, literally believed, and actively used by a group of people in their attempt to understand, explain and control those aspects of life, and reality as a whole, that escape common sense and, more recently, scientific explanation' (2003: 227). In case of spirit manifestation, it is evident that the ideas of people experiencing it escape scientific explanation. Nonetheless, we should not ignore them as they are real for the devotees (see also Schmidt 2016). In the same way I argue also that our subjective experiences of seeing have academic value even if they cannot be proven scientifically. My impressions of different body shapes of mediums alerted me to the physical dimension of spirit manifestation. Spirit manifestations do not happen 'only' within the mind of devotees as the traditional academic interpretation of spirit possession rituals argued. They also take place in a physical space which we can share if we just allow ourselves to see closely. Hence, while my two examples of seeing different body shapes are just based on my subjective experience and not grounded in scientific measurements, they illustrate that even subjective experiences can open a gate into a better understanding of religious experience.

CONCLUSION

I come back to the importance of seeing for anthropologists of religion. Scholars of religion often focus on belief when they study religions, hence on the teachings and worldviews people express when they talk about religions. Anthropologists, on the other side, often focus on the performative aspect of religions: the ceremonies and other practices. In this chapter I argue for a combination of these two approaches, that is based on the notion of experience, i.e. the experience of the researcher. Sight gives us a way to include our experience when attending ceremonies and it is also a bridge to an understanding of the devotees. Instead of focusing on the 'correct' measurements or the 'correct' way of seeing, I highlight the subjective experience of seeing. While acknowledging that what we remember to have seen might sometimes not be correct in a scientific way, these experiences of seeing can further our understanding of religious beliefs and practices outside our own experience.

REFERENCES

Bião, Armindo. (1996) 'Questions posées a la théorie: une approche bahianaise de l'ethnoscénologie,' in Maison des Cultures du Monde (ed.), *La scène et la terre: questions d'ethnoscénologie*. Paris: Babel, pp. 145–152.

Bowie, Fiona. (2012) 'Material and Immaterial Bodies: Ethnographic Reflections on a Trance Séance' (unpublished paper). Available at: https://kcl.academia.edu/FionaBowie/Papers [accessed on 11 December 2012].

Bowie, Fiona. (2016) 'How to Study Religious Experience: Historical and Methodological Reflections on the Study of the Paranormal,' in Schmidt, Bettina E. (ed.), *The Study of Religious Experience: Approaches and Methodologies*. Sheffield, UK: Equinox, pp. 13–32.

Evans-Pritchard, E. E. (1976 [1937]) *Witchcraft, Oracles and Magic among the Azande* (abridged edition). Oxford: Clarendon Press.

Fabian, J. (2002) *Time and the Other: How Anthropology Makes Its Object* (second edition). New York: Columbia University Press.

Fenwick, P. (2001) 'The Neurophysiology of Religious Experience,' in I. Clarke (ed.), *Psychosis and Spirituality*. London: Whurr, pp. 15–26.

Gingrich, Andre. (2005) 'The German-Speaking Countries,' in Barth, Fredrik, Parkin, Robert, Gingrich, Andre and Silverman, Sydel (eds.), *One Discipline, Four Ways: British, German, French, and American Anthropology*. Chicago: University of Chicago Press, pp. 61–156.

Jensen, Adolf Ellegard. (1992 [1951]) *Mythos und Kult bei Naturvölkern*. München: dtv.

Mandressi, Rafaël. (1996) 'L'ethnoscénologie ou la cartographie de terra incognita,' in Maison des Cultures du Monde (ed.), *La scène et la terre: questions d'ethnoscénologie*. Paris: Babel, pp. 91–109.

McCutcheon, R. T. (2012) 'Introduction,' in Martin, C. and McCutcheon, R.T. (eds.), *Religious Experience: A Reader*. Sheffield, UK: Equinox, pp. 1–16.

Münzel, Mark. (1994) 'The Researcher as Shaman: Field-work between Musty Mystification and True Enchantment,' *Anthropology and Ethics*, 3(2), 133–53.

Pradier, Jean-Marie. (1996) 'Ethnoscénologie: La profondeur des émergence,' in Maison des Cultures du Monde (ed.), *La scène et la terre: questions d'ethnoscénologie*. Paris: Babel, pp. 13–41.

Pyysiäinen, I. (2003) *How Religion Works: Towards a New Cognitive Science of Religion*. Leiden: Brill.

Rouget, Gilbert. (1996) 'Questions posées a l'ethnoscénologie,' in Maison des Cultures du Monde (ed.), *La scène et la terre: questions d'ethnoscénologie*. Paris: Babel, pp. 43–53.

Schmidt, Bettina E. (2002) *Karibische Diaspora in New York: Vom ‚Wilden Denken' zur ‚Polyphonen Kultur'*. Berlin: Dietrich Reimer Verlag.

Schmidt, Bettina E. (2008) *Caribbean Diaspora in the USA: Diversity of Caribbean Religions in New York City*. Aldershot, UK: Ashgate.

Schmidt, Bettina E. (2012) '"When the Gods Give Us the Power of Ashé"—Afro-Caribbean Religions as Source for Creative Energy,' in Cusack, C. M. and Norman, A. (eds.), *Handbook of New Religions and Cultural Production* (Brill Handbooks on Contemporary Religion series). The Hague: Brill, pp. 445–61. https://doi.org/10.1163/9789004226487_019

Schmidt, Bettina E. (2014) 'Spirit Possession in Brazil: The Perception of the (Possessed) Body,' *Anthropos*, 109, 135–147.

Schmidt, Bettina E. (2016) *Spirits and Trance in Brazil: An Anthropology of Religious Experience* (Bloomsbury Advances in Religious Studies). London: Bloomsbury.

Sharf, R. H. (1998) 'Experience,' in Taylor, M. (ed.), *Critical Terms for Religious Studies*. Chicago: Chicago University Press, pp. 94–116.

Turner, Edith. (1992) *Experiencing Ritual*. Philadelphia: University of Pennsylvania Press. https://doi.org/10.9783/9780812203981

Turner, Edith. (1993) 'The Reality of Spirits: A Tabooed or Permitted Field of Study,' *Anthropology of Consciousness*, 4(1), 9–12. https://doi.org/10.1525/ac.1993.4.1.9

Dr Bettina E. Schmidt is a cultural anthropologist and currently Professor in the study of religions at the University of Wales Trinity Saint David, and Director of the Alister Hardy Religious Experience Research Centre. She received her doctorate and post-doctorate from the University of Marburg, Germany. Previously she has worked at Marburg University, Oxford University and Bangor University. She was also visiting professor at the City University of New York and visiting scholar at the Pontifícia Universidade Católica de São Paulo. Professor Schmidt is the current President of the British Association for the Study of Religions. She has published extensively on Caribbean and Latin American religions, religious experience, anthropology of religion, identity, cultural theories, gender and migration. Her main fieldwork has been conducted in Mexico, Puerto Rico, Ecuador, New York City and Brazil. She is the author of *Spirits and Trance in Brazil: An Anthropology of Religious Experience* (2016, Bloomsbury), *Caribbean Diaspora in the USA: Diversity of Caribbean Religions in New York City* (2008, Ashgate), *Einführung in die Religionsethnologie* (2008, Reimer Verlag Berlin), and co-editor of *Spirit Possession and Trance: New Interdisciplinary Perspectives* (2010, Continuum) and of the *Handbook of Contemporary Brazilian Religions* (2016, Brill).

Section Three
ILLUMINATION

Chapter 8

Piet Mondrian's Abstraction as a Way of Seeing the Sacred

LIEKE WIJNIA

In January 1909, Dutch painter Piet Mondrian (1872–1944) displayed a painting of a dazzling red mill against a bright yellow sky in the Stedelijk Museum of Amsterdam. Together with two artist friends, Cornelis Spoor and Jan Sluijters, Mondrian had rented several exhibition halls to display their radically modern work. If the artists had not organised it themselves, no museum would have shown their work. While in this particular painting Mondrian intended to convey a specific experience of seeing the world, many of the critics interpreted the painted result in a very literal way. This episode of art history, which will be further discussed below, reflects the key theme of this chapter: the particular mode of seeing that Mondrian meant to convey through his paintings, how his art was meant to encourage this in his viewers, and how the artist's visions differed significantly from the manner in which his contemporaries perceived the artworks.

In this chapter, I will first discuss a figurative painting and an abstract one, respectively from 1908 and 1918. These demonstrate Mondrian's transforming ideas about vision, painterly language and its spiritual potential. Second, selected theoretical writings will shed further light on Mondrian's intentions with his artworks. In his notes and texts, the painter attempted to get at the heart of the interrelationship between his radically abstract language, the modernising world and a spiritually elevated state of mind. Third, to grasp fully the implications of this interrelationship, I explore how Mondrian integrated traditional and modern dynamics of vision in his pictorial and theoretical endeavours.

Overall, I propose a shift in scholarly focus from Mondrian's visual language, which has been dominant in the art-historical paradigm, towards a focus on how he—conceptually and spiritually—viewed the world. As such, it is possible to get a firmer grip on the position of spirituality in his artistic practices. Spirituality is not a temporary engagement or hobby on the side, but located at the heart of Mondrian's work. In Mondrian scholarship, one of the main controversies is whether Mondrian can be characterised as a Theosophical artist and whether his paintings are Theosophical art.[1] Yet, this is not the most fruitful approach to his spirituality. Rather, by means of this chapter, I aim to explore how Mondrian's spirituality is of fundamental importance in the understanding of his artistic practices and his ideas on how art should function in the world. The proposed focus on vision reveals that while Mondrian's spirituality was strongly related to modern urban life, it was also rooted in fundamentally pre-modern ideas on the universality of vision. The paintings served to encourage a spiritually invested mode of seeing the world, for which Mondrian was spiritually developing himself, but to which only a select group of fellow artists, buyers and art lovers was prepared to adhere. It required a change from a mode of seeing dominated by the quest for representation to a mode of seeing which allowed for spiritual elevation.

VISIONS IN PAINT

The painting *Mill: Mill by Sunlight* (1908) is a precursor of Mondrian's later use of primary colours. But at the time of making, the early 1900s, this was not yet an issue for the Dutch painter. After graduating from the art academy in 1895, Mondrian used the genres of urban and landscape painting to explore which style and technique suited him. Over the following years, his primary concern became how to properly capture his viewing of nature on canvas. While he gained a small income from work based on commission, he dedicated his free work to painting natural settings. Evening landscapes were a favourite theme because the setting sun created a mystical atmosphere. Between 1905 and 1908, Mondrian painted many atmospheric evening landscapes in and around the city of Amsterdam.

During those years, he also became acquainted with the vivid and colourful paintings of his Dutch predecessor Vincent van Gogh (1853-1890).

---

1 See for example: Bax (2006: 255-256); Van Paaschen (2017: 7-11); Veen (2017: 29).

Though, or indeed because, for a while it had been forbidden to mention Van Gogh's name at the art academy, Mondrian's young generation of painters had become inspired by his work. *Mill: Mill by Sunlight* demonstrates the way in which Mondrian followed Van Gogh's dynamic use of colour and swift brush strokes. Yet Mondrian used them to a different purpose. While many post-impressionist and later expressionist painters used colour and movement to convey emotional perceptions of a particular setting, for Mondrian colour and texture served the purpose of capturing modes of visual perception itself; not the expression of a state of mind, but the visualisation of a particular way of seeing.

The painting of the red mill against the yellow sky conveys the experience of seeing against brightly shining sunlight, with a shimmering distant horizon. Mondrian translated this onto the canvas by a yellow web of uneven lines and holes. While for the painter this experiment of representing vision in an artistic way meant a radical innovation, contemporary critics, almost unanimously, had no idea what to do with it. Frits Lapidoth described the painting as a mill dripping blood, against a yellow sky with holes like Swiss cheese (Janssen 2007: 122). Jan Kalff wrote that he did not understand the use of colours in the painting at all (Gio 1909). And Conrad Kickert, who in previous pieces had defended Mondrian, now wrote he could follow Mondrian no longer (Janssen 2007: 122).

Only one critic responded positively to the painting, in an article that presented a fierce defence of Mondrian's new, colourful stylistic experiments. This critic was the writer Israël Querido, who published a review of the entire exhibition, but largely focused on Mondrian. Born the same year as Mondrian, Querido was a firm defender of the painter's artistic visions as important expressions of their generation. In his review he consistently calls Mondrian a visionary and describes *Mill: Mill by Sunlight* in lyrical terms.

> What does it represent? The summer day, outside, at its hottest. Again, Mondrian wanted to paint *not* the mill as a pretty mill, not the colour, the sky, the light, trees or atmosphere, as pretty trees, pretty sky colour, but the sensation-moment of the highest glow of the day. (Querido 1909a, cited in De Vries and De Groot 2015: 86)

Because he published his review months after the exhibition had taken place, Querido also incorporated some negative critiques in his defence. One of his targets was the psychiatrist, utopian, and author Frederik van Eeden, who had taken the 1909 exhibition as an opportunity to write an essay about the deterioration in the visual arts. Van Eeden described the colourful work of Mondrian and Sluijters as products of mental illness and 'spiritual decadence' (1909, cited in De Vries and De Groot 2015: 74–79). To Van Eeden, Mondrian especially is a tragic case. The most talented of the three artists in the exhibition has made the deepest fall from grace. By the use of 'raw, barbaric and bright colors,' 'everything that is drawing, composition or technique is lost' (Van Eeden 1909, cited in De Vries and De Groot 2015: 77). He describes Mondrian's work as 'the work of a child – a sick, rowdy child that had a couple of paint tubes at his disposal' (1909, cited in De Vries and De Groot 2015: 77). However, Van Eeden also reassuringly observes that this spiritual decadence may be of temporary nature: 'Such a bewilderment of taste can occur over a short period of time and doesn't necessarily impact a human's soul all too much' (1909, cited in De Vries and De Groot 2015: 77).

Querido forwarded his own review to Mondrian, to which the painter wrote a response. This response was published, with the permission of Mondrian, instead of the concluding part of Querido's three-part review series of the Amsterdam exhibition. It is the earliest published recording of Mondrian's intentions with his art, bordering upon a theoretical text. Notably, he pays special attention to the relationship between his new manner of painting and that of previous generations.

> I find the work of the great masters of the past very beautiful and very grand, but you will agree with me that everything done in our own time must be expressed very differently, even through a different use of technique. I believe that in our period it is definitely necessary that, as far as possible, the paint is applied in pure colors set next to each other in a pointillist or diffuse manner. (…) There are great intrinsic values or truths which remain the same throughout the ages, but form and expression are changing. (Querido 1909b, translated and cited in Welsh 1998: 129)

The notion of intrinsic truths and unchanging values is of crucial importance to understand Mondrian's later development towards abstraction. For Mondrian, the fact that he was searching for a new artistic style that coincided with the rapid development of modern times did not mean the content of what he wanted to express was radically new. On the contrary, it was something inherent, fixed and universal he sought to channel through his art. Mondrian connected this notion of universal values and truths directly to the realm of the spiritual, or, as he also used to call it, 'the occult.' Around these years he was thoroughly invested in the movement of Theosophy. He read many Theosophical texts, described Helena

Blavatsky's *The Secret Doctrine* as 'a true foundation for all things' (Letter, Piet Mondrian to Theo van Doesburg 1919), and saw these types of texts as providing him with gateways to occult knowledge.

Although Mondrian sees a direct relationship between the spiritual knowledge of an artist and the work that this artist produces, he is the first to acknowledge that the wider public is by no means particularly prepared to accept this. That is why, around 1909, he deliberately sticks to painting recognisable subjects: 'For the present at least I shall restrict my work to the customary world of the senses, since that is the world in which we still live. But nevertheless art already can provide a transition to the finer regions, which I call the spiritual realm…' (Querido 1909b, translated and cited in Welsh 1998: 130).

Ten years later, Mondrian's ideas looked very different. In 1918, he produced *Lozenge Composition with Grey Lines*. It is a painting that, as the title indicates, no longer contains any reference to the outside 'customary world of the senses.' Rather, it has become a fully abstract work, in which the painterly tools of line and composition have become the primary characteristics. However, this composition has a closer connection to *Mill: Mill by Sunlight* than it may appear to have on first glance. It requires, indeed, another way of looking. The viewer's vision should not be determined by questions of representation, but rather by a more spiritual, non-representative mode of seeing. Despite its appearance, *Lozenge Composition with Grey Lines* is still very much inspired by a natural phenomenon. As Mondrian wrote in a letter to his friend and *De Stijl* colleague Theo van Doesburg on 1919, it was a 'reconstruction according to the spirit' of a star-filled sky.

This painting is the first in a group of five diamond compositions and, as Marek Wieczorek observes, 'the first work in his oeuvre with straight lines stretching fully from edge to edge, creating an image of totality appropriate for the motif of a starry sky' (2012: 31–32). The construction of the composition is remarkably elementary. Seven horizontal lines and seven vertical lines are placed at even distance from each other. Then, diagonal lines connect the corners of each resulting square. These diagonals are, however, not drawn or painted in one straight line, but connect the corners of the squares one by one. The resulting lines are not completely straight and vary considerably in width and intensity of grey. As a next step, Mondrian began to fill in the resulting small triangles, which also have various sizes and forms. Just as the lines vary in grey and black tones, the small triangles vary in tones of white, beige and light grey. The result is visually astonishing.

This seemingly static raster turns out to be an intricate interplay of lines and shades. Especially at the points where the diagonals, horizontals and verticals meet, the eyes seem to notice a flickering movement. If the viewer then wants to focus on the intersection of movement, the flickering swiftly moves elsewhere in the composition. The embodiment of movement in the pictorial surface makes the composition simultaneously endlessly deep and undeniably flat. As Hans Janssen observes, this is a similar experience to looking at the starry sky at night. From earth, the sky appears to be flat and repetitive, while it is at the same time endlessly far away and impossible to grasp (Janssen 2016: 614). The incorporation of this dual sense of perception, resulting in the effect of shimmering, makes *Lozenge Composition in Grey Lines* a direct successor to *Mill: Mill by Sunlight*. In the ultimate flatness of this entirely abstract composition, Mondrian had found a dynamic way of conveying a visual perception, as he had actually experienced in the visible world. By translating the essence of his perception in paint onto a canvas, he aimed to encourage a similar engagement in his viewers. I would argue that it is this translation process (from viewing and experiencing to a painterly composition) in which the spiritual qualities of Mondrian's artistic approach are invested.

In a matter of ten years, Mondrian had found a pictorial language with which he could capture and convey his visionary ideas. These were not necessarily visions of an otherworldly spiritual realm. Rather, his visions regarded a spiritually invested mode of seeing the world around him, the rapidly modernising world he was living in. An example of this mode of seeing can be found already in 1909 when Mondrian described to a journalist how he would convey a dance evening on a canvas. In an article ten years later, the journalist recalls his answer: 'Well, I abstract her in vertical and horizontal lines' ('Hollandsche Kunstenaarskring iii' 1909).[2] He approached this dance evening in the same manner he approached landscapes, with the aim to uncover its fundamental structures. Mondrian approached the visible world around him in the artistic instruments of colour, form and composition, which he had at his disposal as a painter.

VISIONS IN TEXT

In conjunction with his experiments with painterly instruments and visual language, Mondrian kept notebooks and began to express the

---

2 Hans Janssen (2016: 614, note 40) suggests the anonymous author of this piece to be Augusta de Meester-Obreen.

desire to publish theoretical texts. His writings shed further light on how he regarded the language of abstraction as the embodiment of a spiritual mode of seeing. The 1909 letter to Querido had originally been written as personal correspondence. Mondrian frequently corresponded with family, fellow artists, and (potential) collectors and benefactors. He was, however, very adamant about the destiny of his letters. More than once he instructed those at the receiving end to destroy the letters after reading, because the contents were deemed strictly personal, even when he wrote about his art or other professional matters.[3]

Mondrian maintained a different attitude towards his theoretical texts. In addition to his personal sketchbooks, which he also used as notebooks, he wrote many texts from about 1916 onwards. He had fellow artists read and provide feedback on these texts, and intended them to become accessible to a wider audience. Yet, more than once his attempts at publishing failed. The first extensive text was titled *Neo-Plasticism in Pictorial Art*, written between late 1914 and 1918. Originally intended to be published as one book, Mondrian eventually accepted the offer by Van Doesburg to have the text published in instalments in the new modern art magazine *De Stijl*.

This magazine was launched with Van Doesburg as editor-in-chief in November 1917 as a platform for avant-garde artists. Not only painters, but also likeminded architects, sculptors, designers and artists in other disciplines were invited to join. *De Stijl* was to become synonymous with a breakdown of the traditional hierarchy in artistic disciplines. It promoted a vision in which painters, architects and sculptors should collaborate to create works of art in which each contribution was equally valuable, and valued. While this approach made for an innovative discussion platform on paper, in practice the ideal of interdisciplinary collaboration was cause for disagreement more than once.

Already around the time he painted *Mill: Mill by Sunlight*, Mondrian was keenly interested in the latest philosophical trends. He described the impact of philosophical knowledge, which he saw as an early stage leading to spiritual knowledge, on artistic practices:

> It seems to me that you too recognize the important relationship between philosophy and art, and it is exactly this relationship which most painters deny. The great masters grasp it unconsciously, but I believe that a painter's

---

3 This is also the reason why very few letters written to Mondrian have survived. As he expected from his correspondents, he almost consistently destroyed the letters he received. Still, many at the receiving end of his letters did not adhere to his request. See Bax (2006: 254–255, note 153).

conscious spiritual knowledge will have a much greater influence upon his art, and that it is merely a weakness in him—or a lack of genius—should this spiritual knowledge be harmful to his art. (Querido 1909b, translated and cited in Welsh 1998: 129–130).

In addition to the act of painting, another fruitful way of cultivating this spiritual knowledge for Mondrian was writing. In a letter of September 1919 to Willy Wentholt, Mondrian declared that 'writing is a great way of expressing myself.' In an interview several years later he reinforces this point: 'It is hard to explain the intention of my paintings. In the works themselves I have expressed things as well as I could. (...) The reverse side, what remains unspoken, can be better set forth in an article' (Van Loon 1922). In the final years of his life, after he fled to the United States due to the Second World War, he was still very much occupied with writing texts to support his artworks and reach new audiences. Remarkably, when he moved to a new country he would immediately adopt the English language for his texts. His English was not as up to standard as his French was. In New York, his friend Charmion von Wiegand offered help editing and revising the texts written between 1941 and 1944.

Mondrian soon recognised that a radical new art could not be fully explained with the language that was also used to discuss the more traditional, established art forms. This was a wider trend throughout Europe, as historian Guido van Hengel has demonstrated (Van Hengel 2018: 75). Many utopian thinkers and writers coined neologisms in an attempt to capture the changing Zeitgeist, particularly the crucial importance of the inner life in the rapidly changing world. One of them was the previously mentioned Frederik van Eeden, who was one of The Netherland's most famous (and notorious) utopian thinkers. His writings and initiatives (after the example of the American philosopher and transcendentalist Henri David Thoreau, he founded a living community called Walden in the Dutch town of Laren) were all attempts to battle spiritual decadence, as Van Eeden identified it in Mondrian's paintings of 1908. Although their visions of the future looked significantly different, both men strived to contribute to the frameworks and conditions for a new era, which expressed a new spirit, and both needed a new language in order to give expression to these aims.

With the 1917 publication of *Neo-Plasticism in Pictorial Art*, Mondrian introduced the term with which he characterised his abstract visual language. The word Neo-Plasticism in the later English translation originated as the Dutch *Nieuwe Beelding*. The term *beelding* did not, and still does not, exist in the Dutch language. Mondrian seems to have borrowed the term from the writings of philosopher and theologian Matthieu Schoenmaekers, who used it in relation to his theory of metaphysical mathematics (Blotkamp 2001 [1994]: 111). Mondrian got acquainted with Schoenmaekers during the years of the First World War, when both took up residence in Laren. The word is derived from terms such as *afbeelding*, meaning representation, and *verbeelding*, meaning imagination. As these two terms are used in reference to established art traditions, Mondrian felt he had to come up with a new word to characterise the radically new turn he wanted his art to represent. He was after an art that was independent of all that had happened before. In continuous discussion with his fellow artists of *De Stijl*, Mondrian came to use the term *beelding*. It is a term independent of references to representation or imagination, but instead an art that functioned and existed independently of (figurative) traditions. Not directly referencing anything visible in the outside world, Mondrian's art was to embody the relationships of which that world essentially consisted: not visible to the eye, but structurally present behind visible reality.

This was an utterly spiritual approach to art, for which Mondrian based his thinking on various sources.[4] However, his writing emerged in strong symbiosis with his artistic practices, as illustrated in a statement by Von Wiegand: 'the paintings come first and the theory comes from the paintings' (Rowell 1971: 82). The materiality of painting formed a restriction in the expression of something fundamentally immaterial. As such, Mondrian placed his art in between the earthly, natural domain and the spiritual, divine domain. This is why he called his abstract paintings *abstract-real*. 'Because she exists between the absolute-abstract and the natural, concrete-real. She is not so abstract as thought-abstraction and she is not so real as the material reality. She is aesthetically living plasticism: the appearance in which the one is present in the other' (Mondrian 1918a: 29–31).

In his thinking, Mondrian consistently seeks the balance between opposites: natural-spiritual, objective-subjective, universal-particular, abstract-real, etc. He acknowledged that his paintings could not establish a fully spiritually elevated state on their own. Yet, the artworks could function as precursors to his envisioned abstract way of engaging with the visible

---

4 In his early writing years, Mondrian found important sources in the work of Neo-Hegelian philosopher Gerard Bolland; theologian and philosopher Matthieu Schoenmaekers; founder of the Theosophical movement Helena Blavatsky; and founder of Anthroposophy Rudolf Steiner.

world. Hence, in order to fully grasp what Mondrian wanted to express with his art, it is not only important to see his radical artistic innovations, but also to join him in a new understanding of the world. For Mondrian, abstraction did not only concern art, it concerned life in its entirety. To emphasise this view of the world, he coined a new word: *ziening*. This is the visionary equivalent of *beelding*, which could be loosely translated as *visioning*. To Mondrian, there were different gradations of *ziening*, but ultimately if one was capable of objective *ziening*, it meant one was able to view the world in the way Mondrian expressed this worldview in his art. He maintained this idea throughout his life, with the telling title of a 1942 text: *Towards the True Vision of Reality*.

Mondrian saw his new pictorial instruments, the fully abstract visual language, as witness to a new *ziening*. His art is no longer about what it represents, but about the harmony and balance achieved by means of pictorial instruments (Mondrian 1917a: 2–6). This requires a new mode of vision, which he as artist was keen to develop.

> The artistic temperament, the *aesthetic* vision, acknowledges the style; the everyday vision, on the contrary, sees this [neither] in art nor in nature. Everyday vision is the vision of the individual, which cannot elevate beyond the individual. As long as the material is viewed in an individual manner, the style cannot be seen. As such everyday vision obstructs all art. She does not *want* style in art, she desires the detailed image. However, the artist *wants* and *searches* [for] style: that is his struggle. (Mondrian 1917b, pp. 13–18)

Many art historians primarily focus on the notion of *beelding*, with the aim to grasp the artistic significance of Mondrian's abstraction. However, if we are to better understand the elementary role of spirituality in his artistic practices, the notion of *ziening* is essential. In his linguistic inventiveness, Mondrian even combined the two notions into the term of *beeldend zien*. This embeds the pictorial instruments of line and colour in the spiritual mode of viewing. I would argue that this *beeldend zien* is not only a theory of art but needs to be understood as worldview—as a spiritual engagement with the world as well as with existential questions about the future of that world. In 1919, Mondrian wrote, 'The pure *Beeldend zien* has to build a new society, like in the arts it has built a new plastic—a society of equal dualities between the material and the spiritual, a society of balanced relationships' (Mondrian 1919–1920, cited in Veen 2017: 154). For Mondrian, his new art was intrinsically rooted in a vision of a new world.

Beyond relating his paintings to the latest developments in the international art world, Mondrian felt there was a larger social and spiritual urgency to his work. This social urgency was strongly connected to Mondrian's life in urban contexts like Amsterdam, Paris, London and New York (Mondrian 1919–1920, cited in Veen 2017: 156). Yet, his spirituality, while drawn from and oriented toward this modern urban life, has notably pre-modern foundations. His ideals about a spiritual state of mind, and the role his art could play in potentially encouraging this, were rooted in essentially traditional ideas about vision. This paradox of linking pre-modern and modern perceptions is well illustrated by Mondrian's own acknowledgement of the discrepancy between his radically new abstract language and the unchanging, timeless truth he tried to convey with it.

(PRE-)MODERN VISIONS

Mondrian advocated spirituality through vision, which he encouraged in people by having them look at his paintings. Yet his spiritual claims were often conceived of as rigid, strict and dogmatic. This dogmatic perception was more linked to Mondrian's use of limited visual elements (horizontals, verticals, primary colours) rather than to the content of the spiritual claims (De Gruyter 1942, cited in Rijnders 2016: 248–249). For many, the unchanging, traditional, timeless universality Mondrian claimed to convey went over their heads. Essentially, in order to move forward in creating a new art for the future, Mondrian attempted to look back as far as he could. Historian Hermann von der Dunk has argued how it seems to be a fundamental aspect of modernity to return to the past (2000: 375). This is a tendency that can be recognised in various modern art movements, from the Pre-Raphaelites in Britain to the French Surrealists. While the latter looked to the uninhibited and seemingly untrained pictorial language of medieval artists, the former carried their heroes of the past in the very name of their movement. For Mondrian, the engagement with the past concerned the notion of vision—and the values attributed to vision.

To Mondrian this return to the past was simultaneously a turn to the future, or everlasting, which he conveys via a parallel with religion:

> All religions have the same primordial content: they only differ in form. The *form* is its external representation: this form is something indispensible for the expression of the primordial principles. (...) Hence, form is dependent on the *time* and on the degree of *development* of mankind. This means that the *form* can never be the same all the time. Including the *form* in art. (Mondrian 1914, cited in Veen 2017: 74)

This paradox of the old and the new was a recurring theme that he felt needed explanation. In part six of *Neoplasticism in Pictorial Art*, Mondrian admitted, 'Seemingly it is little *modern* to base oneself on an old truth in order to shed light on the reasonableness of the new' (Mondrian 1918c, cited in Veen 2017: 98). He took the opportunity of this text to write a defence of the reasoning behind his newfound ideas about abstraction. The strongest argument was, to him, the notion of universality. He continued that it was: '[s]eemingly so, because the new is not very different from another *appearance* of the universal truth, which is unchanging' (Mondrian 1918c, cited in Veen 2017: 98).

In order to grasp these universal, unchanging principles, a new mode of seeing was required, first for the artist producing the paintings, and subsequently for viewers. To get a sense of the elements from which Mondrian constructed his ideas about vision, Jonathan Crary's analysis of dramatic changes in the organisation of vision over the course of the nineteenth century is useful. Crary explored how the early nineteenth-century model of vision underwent a radical shift. This shift does not, as often argued in art-historical discourse, constitute of a range of artists reinventing the visual arts, leading to Impressionism and post-Impressionism, and the invention of photography (Crary 1990: 4). In tracing the development of vision, Crary proposes to move beyond the study of selected artistic practices, by looking at the 'phenomenon of the observer' (1990: 5).

Crary argues, 'Vision and its effects are always inseparable from the possibilities of an observing subject who is both the historical product and the site of certain practices, techniques, institutions, and procedures of subjectification' (1990: 5). This leads to a definition of the observer being someone who 'sees within a prescribed set of possibilities, one who is embedded in a system of conventions and limitations' (1990: 6). It is precisely the identified changes in this system of conventions and limitations that are of interest in the study of Mondrian's envisioned mode of *ziening* and its perception by a broader public.

Crary analyses the dramatic shift for the observer by means of optical devices. He sees 'the camera obscura as paradigmatic of the dominant status of the observer in the seventeenth and eighteenth centuries,' while in the nineteenth century the stereoscope becomes of primary importance (Crary 1990: 8). The crucial implications of these devices for the status of the observer are that the camera obscura was thought to establish an objective perception, reliable and truthful; yet, with the introduction of new optical instruments like the stereoscope, vision became increasingly tied to the body. The more embodied experience of vision led it to be perceived as individual, subjective and open to misperception and flaws.

In Crary's analysis, there is a very clear development from one phase to the next. However, I propose that Mondrian's ideas about vision can only be understood if these two phases are regarded as intertwined. Mondrian's visual language of abstraction was undeniably innovative, radical and modern. It is the type of visual language to which individuals can relate in a very personal, subjective manner. Yet, what he wanted to express with this pictorial language was of timeless, unchanging and objective nature. As generations of artists had done before him in finding modes of expression for religious principles, Mondrian attempted to grasp an underlying, invisible essence that he discussed in terms of the spiritual. He regarded organised religion, its imagery and symbolism, as institutional forms for conveying this underlying spiritual essence. With his art, he offered an alternative form, one that was suitable for the world of his time, and that of the future as he envisioned it. As he formulated it, 'by seeing in a manner of *beelding* we improve as it were our regular visual *ziening* – and this way we relate the individual to the universal: that is how the pure *beeldend* vision unites us with the universal' (Mondrian 1919–1920, in Veen 2017: 152).

CONCLUSION

Some contemporaries recognised the spiritual significance of Mondrian's visual language early on. Theo van Doesburg was one of them, when he wrote in 1915, before he and Mondrian had met in person:

> From a spiritual point of view, this work is superior to everything else. It gives an impression of repose, the passivity of the soul. (…) To reduce the means to a minimum and then present an artistic impression of such purity with nothing more than some white paint on a white canvas and a few horizontal and plumb lines – this is exceptional. (Van Doesburg 1915: 11)

Yet, as illustrated above, most fellow artists and critics could not follow the artist in his pictorial development.

Mondrian was very concerned about his contemporaries misunderstanding his art. This occasionally resulted in frustration and is a recurring theme in his theoretical texts. Mondrian always had one eye on the future, where humans would be more attuned to higher sensory dimensions. In the meantime, his paintings served to encourage people at least to try to develop their spiritual sensibilities. In a sketchbook of 1914, Mondrian noted, 'The artist intuitively sees in a more spiritual manner than ordinary humans: that is why he sees reality more beautifully, which makes his art good for ordinary humans. However, the artist-human requires another artist who can see more beautifully than him, and this human has the need for an abstract art' (Mondrian 1914, cited in Veen 2017: 69). Although the majority of his contemporaries may not have fully grasped his art, Mondrian argued that even those who misunderstood it still had an intuition for the sublime. In a letter of 1932 to Louk Hoyack, he called this intuition 'the divine in mankind.' For Mondrian, the notion of intuition was strongly related to spiritual attunement, which in turn would be evolutionarily developed. The time-span of almost twenty years between the sketchbook and the letter demonstrates how this question of the spiritual, its visual expression and its public perception, remained themes of importance.

Mondrian envisioned a future in which people would be spiritually able to experience the world's fundamental structures. In all his paintings and texts, the notion of vision has a crucial position. They are about multiple experiences of seeing, grounded in subjective and objective dynamics of vision combined. Rather than representing another, higher spiritual dimension, I would argue that Mondrian's paintings can be regarded as ultimately representing and encouraging a spiritually invested mode of engaging with this world. To Mondrian, his paintings embodied a 'living reality,' and he invited people to engage with them in this manner (1918b, cited in Veen 2017: 96). As such, Mondrian explained:

> the abstract-real painting can also be *art* to those who have not yet fully developed the new sense of time. The spiritual content can be *experienced* subconsciously. But—generally—the visual language is in the way of complete appreciation of the work of art. The visual language is too new, too unusual, when the mind is not pre-conceived with the idea of the true visual manifestation of the universal. (Mondrian 1918b, cited in Veen 2017: 96)

In this chapter, I have aimed to unveil Mondrian's paradoxical endeavour of combining pre-modern and modern modes of seeing in the encouragement of spiritual visions within his viewers. The painter seemed to be fully aware of this discrepancy, but nevertheless pursued it throughout his artistic career. As I have argued, this discrepancy turned out to be a persistent feature in the public reception of his art. Many critics were not prepared to take up the challenge to move beyond the surface in their own vision, and remained at the level of literally interpreting the pictorial language of the paintings. This challenge still constitutes a large presence in research and exhibition practices. In response, my proposed shift in scholarly focus from Mondrian's abstract visual language (*beelding*) to its visionary equivalent (*ziening*), could serve as a relevant step in the perception of his art as a 'living reality,' as an embodiment of Mondrian's worldview.

As such, Mondrian paved the way for many artists of coming generations, especially those working with vision as their primary material. While Mondrian had a life-long commitment to paint and canvas, others after him had new means and methods to impact the audience's vision. In, for example, performance, installation and land art, the participation of audience members has become quintessential in the functioning and completion of the works of art. This engagement is often described in terms of spirituality and transcendence. Mondrian was already concerned with these participatory and experiential levels, but got stuck mediating between objective and subjective modes of vision. Generations of artists who followed fully embraced vision's modern qualities of subjectivity and embodiment, resulting in again radically new, spiritually engaged bodies of art.

BIBLIOGRAPHY

Primary Sources

Gio (Jan Kalff). (1909) 'Kunst en wetenschappen. C. Spoor, P. Mondriaan, J. Sluijters,' *Algemeen Handelsblad*, 14 January, Avondblad, Tweede Blad, 7.
'Hollandsche Kunstenaarskring iii,' *Nieuwe Rotterdamsche Courant*, 17 March 1909, Avondblad A1.
Letter, Piet Mondrian to Theo van Doesburg. (1919) The Hague: RKD—Netherlands Institute for Art History, Archive Theo and Nelly van Doesburg Archives, 18 April.
Letter, Piet Mondrian to Willy Wentholt. (1919) The Hague: RKD—Netherlands Institute for Art History, 6 September.
Letter, Piet Mondrian to Louk Hoyack. (1932) The Hague: RKD—Netherlands Institute for Art History, Archive Louk and Ella Hoyack, 27 June.
Mondrian, Piet. (1914) 'Kunst en Realiteit,' cited in Veen (2017: 68–69).
Mondrian, Piet. (1917a) 'De nieuwe beelding in de schilderkunst,' *De Stijl*, 1(1), October, 2–6.
Mondrian, Piet. (1917b) 'De nieuwe beelding in de schilderkunst,' *De Stijl*, 1(2), December, 13–18.
Mondrian, Piet. (1918a) 'De nieuwe beelding in de schilderkunst,' *De Stijl*, 4(3), January, 29–31.

Mondrian, Piet. (1918b) 'IV. De Redelijkheid der Nieuwe Beeldin,' March, cited in Veen (2017: 94-98).
Mondrian, Piet. (1918c) 'VI. De Redelijkheid der Nieuwe Beelding (Vervolg),' April, cited in Veen (2017: 98-102).
Mondrian, Piet. (1919-1920) 'Natuurlijke en abstracte realiteit. Slot 3e toneel,' *De Stijl*, cited in Veen (2017: 151-154).
Van Doesburg, Theo. (1915) 'Kunst-Kritiek,' *Eenheid*, 6(283), 11.
Van Loon, Henri. (1922) 'Bij Piet Mondriaan,' *Nieuwe Rotterdamsche Courant*, 23 March, Avondblad B.

Secondary Sources

Bax, Marty. (2006) *Het Web der Schepping, Theosofie en Kunst in Nederland, Van Lauweriks tot Mondriaan*. Amsterdam: SUN.
Blotkamp, Carel. (2001 [1994]) *Mondrian: The Art of Destruction*. Chicago: University of Chicago Press.
Crary, Jonathan. (1990) *Techniques of the Observer, On Vision and Modernity in the Nineteenth Century*. Cambridge, MA, London: MIT Press.
De Gruyter, W. Jos. (1942) 'Piet Mondriaan zeventig jaar,' *Het Vaderland. Staat—en Letterkundig Nieuwsblad*, 6 maart.
De Vries, Jan and De Groot, Marijke (eds.) (2015) *Van Vuurwerk Sintels Maken. Kunstkritiek en moderne kunst, 1905-1925*. Rotterdam: NAI Uitgevers, pp. 74-79.
Janssen, Hans. (2007) *Mondriaan in het Gemeentemuseum*. Zwolle: Waanders.
Janssen, Hans. (2016) *Piet Mondriaan. Een nieuwe kunst voor een ongekend leven. Een biografie*. Amsterdam: Hollands Diep.
Querido, Israël. (1909a) 'Een schilder-studie. Spoor, Mondriaan en Sluijters,' *De Controleur*, 29 May.
Querido, Israël. (1909b) 'Van menschen en dingen. Een schilders-studie. Spoor, Mondrian, en Sluijters. Piet Mondriaan. (slot),' *De Controleur*, 20(1004), 23 October, second quire, no page number.
Rijnders, Mieke (ed.) (2016) *Realisme in Nederland, Critici kiezen positie. 1925-1945*. Rotterdam: NAI010 Uitgevers.
Rowell, Margit. (1971) 'Interview with Charmion von Wiegand (20 June 1971),' *Piet Mondrian Centennial Exhibition* (Exhibition Catalogue). New York: Solomon R. Guggenheim Museum, pp. 77-86.
Van Eeden, Frederik. (1909) 'Gezondheid en verval in kunst, (naar aanleiding der tentoonstelling Spoor—Mondriaan—Sluijters)', *Op de Hoogte. Maandschrift voor in de huiskamer*, 6(2), 79-85.
Van Hengel, Guido. (2018) *De Zieners. Visioenen uit een verloren Europa*. Amsterdam: Prometheus.
Van Paaschen, Jacqueline. (2017) *Mondriaan en Steiner, Wegen naar nieuwe beelding*. The Hague: Komma/d'jonge Hond.
Veen, Louis (ed.) (2017) *Piet Mondrian, The Complete Writings*. Leiden: Primavera Press.

Von der Dunk, Hermann W. (2000) *De verdwijnende hemel: Over de cultuur van Europa in de twintigste eeuw*, part 1. Amsterdam: Meulenhoff.
Welsh, Robert P. (ed.) (1998) *Catalogue raisonné of the Naturalistic Works (until early 1911), I. Blaricum*, Paris: V+K Publishing/Inmerc, Editions Cercle d'Art.
Wieczorek, Marek. (2012) 'Mondrian's First Diamond Composition,' in Crowther, Paul and Wünsche, Isabel (eds.), *Meanings of Abstract Art. Between Nature and Theory*. London: Routledge, pp. 30–46.

Paintings Discussed

Piet Mondrian [1872–1944], *Mill: Mill by Sunlight*, 1908. Oil on canvas, 114 × 87 cm. Kunstmuseum Den Haag.
Piet Mondrian [1872–1944], *Lozenge Composition with Grey Lines*, 1918. Oil on canvas, 84.5 × 84.5 cm. Kunstmuseum Den Haag: https://www.kunstmuseum.nl/en/collection/composition-grid-3-lozenge-composition-grey-lines?origin=gm?origin=gm

Lieke Wijnia is curator of modern and contemporary collections at Museum Catharijneconvent in Utrecht, and a fellow with the Centre for Religion and Heritage at the University of Groningen. After obtaining MA degrees in heritage studies at Utrecht University and art history at the Courtauld Institute of Art, she defended her PhD thesis cum laude at Tilburg University in 2016, on perceptions of the sacred at Festival Musica Sacra Maastricht. She recently published *Beyond the Return of Religion: Art and the Postsecular* (Brill, 2018). Her essay collection on the quest for the sacred in art museums was honoured by the Teylers Theological Society with their 2017 gold medal. Her research on Piet Mondrian's spirituality was honoured with the inaugural Jeffrey Rubinoff Sculpture Park Postdoctoral Award in 2018. That award allowed her to produce the chapter for this volume.

Chapter 9

Sacred Landscapes, New Conversations: Paul Nash's Visionary Paintings of the Wittenham Clumps

MOLLY KADY

Paul Nash (1889–1946) studied at the Slade School, London in 1910–1911 and held his first one-man show in 1912. He served as an official war artist in both World Wars, and developed an asthmatic condition from exposure to shellfire in 1917, which resulted in his early death in 1946. Some of his work indicates the influence of abstract art and surrealism. As well as being a war artist he was a photographer, writer and designer of applied art. He is most famous for his landscape paintings and is considered to be one of the finest artists of the first half of the twentieth century. This chapter focuses on his landscape paintings, in particular three of the many depictions he created of the Wittenham Clumps, Oxfordshire.

From his earliest artistic representations of the Wittenham Clumps, Nash challenged his audience to envision what was not there. He tested their immediate awareness and sensory appetite to search for the unseen. Nash's depictions of this landscape are currently enjoying a revival of interest and continue to evoke the presence of the elusive persons and forces he saw and identified in his landscapes.

The Clumps (**Figure 9.1**), two mammiform hills, two miles northwest of Wallingford in the Sinodun Range, Oxfordshire, have a fascinating history as a Neolithic burial site that was later occupied by a Roman army. However, Nash's landscape paintings of the Wittenham Clumps offer viewers a different way of looking at the site. As nature and objects within the natural world became increasingly important to him, Nash returned physically and pictorially to the Clumps many times. Defining his work as

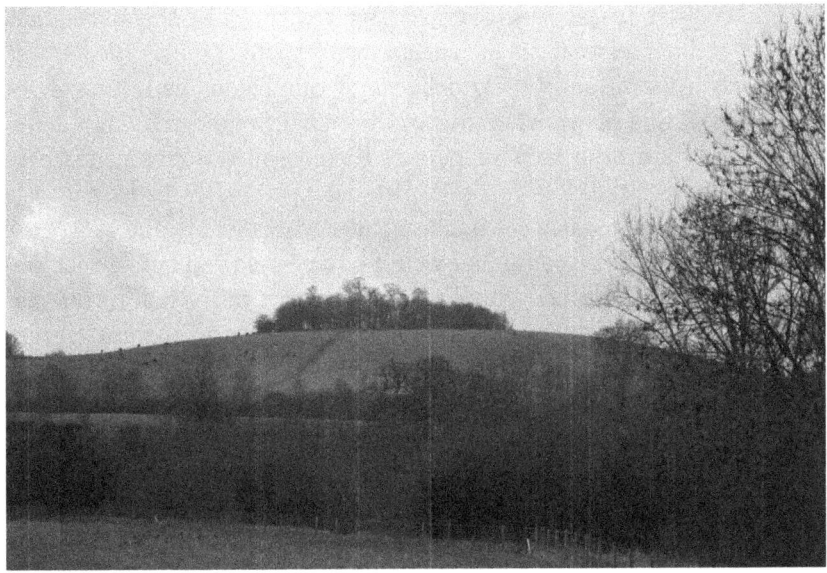

Figure 9.1 The Wittenham Clumps, December, 2017. Photo by Graham Harvey. © Molly Kady.

spiritual was a problem for Nash. However, by reading James Frazer and William Wordsworth he gained an understanding of their ontology which guided him to an ontological understanding of his own work, enabling him to locate the pagan and animist essence that imbues his landscape paintings.

The use of the terms spirit or spiritual are problematic even today but as Graham Harvey claims, 'It might just be a way in which some people try to convey an idea about their personal relationship with trees, animals, rivers or ancestors that others consider inanimate and inert' (Harvey 2013a: 4). David Shorter also argues that these terms are misleading as they deny clarity and are so overused as to cover almost every human experience to the stage where they mean absolutely nothing: 'Spiritual fails to mean anything reliable due to the range of meanings the term has held throughout various languages and historical eras' (Shorter 2016: 434). It is more helpful to assert that Nash was experiencing a vitalist response to his world, commensurate with his earliest encounters with being in nature (Nash 1988 [1949]: 35), meaning he was fully and intensely alive to the vital principle of all life. His work on the Clumps is redolent with what Charlene Spretnak calls 'participatory, engaged consciousness' (Spretnak 1999: 136). His images of the Clumps indicate how he rejected the notion that 'modern society lives on top of nature' (Spretnak 1999: 3).

This chapter traces Nash's visual engagement with the Wittenham Clumps and argues that his pagan/animist response to his vision of the Clumps is a useful and timely analysis of this landscape. Although he refused to define his conviction about the English landscape in a definitively Christian or otherwise overtly theological way, his concern to address vitalist issues like 'respecting all our relations in the living world to make the world a much better place,' clearly vocalised by Harvey (2016), is a pagan/animist response and would be accepted today as a religious response: '"Nature" can refer to the unity of all that exists, rooting humans in the wider cosmic community and sometimes requiring humans to relinquish separatist ambitions' (Harvey 2016: 363).

Nash's awareness of there being more to the landscape than was visible to the eye was a sensation that originated in his childhood (Nash 1988 [1949]: 36). As a child, he engaged with the personalities of trees that changed with the seasons and light; at times appearing bewitched, at others enchanted whilst 'guarding the threshold of a domain' (Nash 1988 [1949]: 35). By adulthood, the responses that the natural world drew from him were already firmly encompassed within his artistic agenda. His involvements in both World Wars, where he witnessed landscapes blasted and devastated, clearly depicted in his lithograph, *Void of War* (1918) and his most well-known work, *Menin Road* (1918–19), cut deeply into his psyche.[1] This destruction alerted him even more keenly to the importance of responding to the conversational voice of the natural world, which had been ignored. The first letter Nash received from Gordon Bottomley in 1910 encouraged him to allow his 'insight and vision' to produce art that reinstated the sacrality of landscape that the obliterating forces of war destroyed (Nash 1988 [1949]: 85).

Although most of Nash's work omits human activity, the Clumps, as an ancient burial mound, is saturated with human presence. Roger Cardinal argues that Nash was instinctively drawn to places like the Clumps because of their natural configuration and allure (Cardinal 2016 [1989]: 7). However, as Nash himself claimed, he painted what he saw with an interior view of the landscape he envisioned (Nash 1988 [1949]: 80). His portrayals of the Clumps, before and after the wars, reinvested a sacred status in this site. Having already abandoned what he perceived as outdated notions of religion, Nash looked for different ways of responding to the Clumps' appeal.

---

1 Nash, P. (1918) *Void of War*, lithograph on paper, 48.9 × 57.4 cm, Imperial War Museum, London; Nash, P. (1918–19) *Menin Road*, oil, 182.8 × 317.5 cm, Imperial War Museum, London.

Nash explored and reworked this landscape many times to understand its power (Hall 1996: 19). This was not to gain new ideas but to listen to the landscape and allow it to speak for itself as it did in his boyhood. He recalls: 'I reached at last the sweet Alderbourne talking in its limpid tones in the still of the night, for talk it did, most convincingly, nor was its voice the only one I could hear...' (Nash 1988 [1949]: 78). Trees were personages, rivers and streams spoke to him. Andrew Causey claims that it was Nash's way of painting that made inanimate things speak for him (Causey 1975 [1951]: 6). However, according to Nash's own perspective, he painted as he did because the landscape spoke to him from its own power and personality. Nash did not see himself investing these qualities into his art: they were ever-present in the landscape he visualised. It is primarily this engagement with the personages of the landscape, I argue, that is a religious act. From all these relationships Nash's collective receptivity to all of nature was nourished.

Returning to the Clumps in later life, he was drawn to celebrating new conversations about being in the world and expressing his reciprocal relationship with it. He experienced this in places where he felt situated in 'meditative stillness [with a sensation of] having arrived [and being able to engage with] certain values, already perceptible within himself' (Cardinal 2016 [1989]: 13). Nash sat among stones and trees in the landscape to emphasise his personhood within it. With reference to debates about ontology, Harvey claims: 'To be a person is to act with, among and towards others' (Harvey 2005: 227; also see 2013b). In this manner, Nash engages with Earth's ecological community.

Nash's pictorial and physical interactions within the sacred space referred to as the Clumps honed his artistic tools for interrogating a world beyond human sight. Following Nash's vision, viewers are challenged and channelled into seeing the world and perhaps the 'unseen' differently. Causey suggests that Nash was inferring rather than positing unseen presences or personages in the landscape, and that may have been a more acceptable response at the time. He goes on to argue that Nash made animate and inanimate things speak for him in his depictions (Causey 1975 [1951]: 6). To refer to Nash's landscape art as the realm of the dream world is misleading if in doing so it denies the psychological forces at play within Nash. However, Causey argues that Nash's boundaries between the dream and reality are porous (Causey 2013: 26). Like James Laver, I support a clear and robust claim that Nash was penetrating the physical and encountering the other (Laver 1975 [1951]: 17), whilst going further by suggesting that the other spoke to him. Viewers need to be prepared for the psychological maelstrom Nash lays before them, as we do not generally see the personalities with which places are charged. Leonard Robinson argues that all of Nash's work mirrored the psychological forces within himself (Robinson 1997: xxv), but his work has the ability to lead the observant into his vision. Nash may have found it difficult to put into words exactly what it was he saw in certain places but his visual narrative, as well as indications from his writings, give us an insight into his ontological view of landscapes.

Particular places had very strong personal involvement and special significance for him. In *Outline* he wrote, 'this tree guarded the threshold of a domain, which, for me, was like hallowed ground...there are places, just as there are people and objects and works of art, whose relationship of parts creates a mystery, an enchantment, which cannot be analysed' (Nash 1988 [1949]: 35). In a letter to Mercia Oakley in 1911, Nash revealed his acute sense of the relationship between the past and the present. He commented on how strange and enchanted the Clumps were. He saw them as legendary and haunted by old gods (cited by Jenkins et al. 2010: 37). Nash was enchanted by a world beyond that which is experienced directly. He returned to the Clumps many times to discover their 'hidden relationships' (Causey 1975 [1951]: 5). Laver has argued that 'He soared around and above the Wittenham Clumps in the dream-like flight he sought in his childhood' (Laver 1975 [1951]: 12). I argue that it was the inner life of this location that captivated him: It was, as he said, 'Always the inner life of the subject rather than its characteristic lineaments which appealed to me... the secret of a place lies there for everybody to find, though not, perhaps, to understand' (Nash 1988 [1949]: 36).

Nash recognised the Clumps as a place 'brimming with concealed significance and the path representing the journey leading to it' (Sloan 2017: 62). A recurring trope in his work is pathways, pathways through woodland and arching trees; features that are attached to his personal involvement in a place. In a letter to Gordon Bottomley, Nash wrote, 'I sincerely love and worship trees and know they are people' (cited by Bertram 1955: 42). In 1909, in an unpublished poem dedicated to Mercia Oakley, he wrote about trees as 'dreaming, swooning in sleepful wakefulness.... An encyclopaedia of the ancient past found in trees' (cited by Causey 2013: 28). A childhood experience of a pathway leading through a spinney and passing a stream was imprinted on his memory; the mood and details of a landscape clearly recalled from a dream. Shadowed aspects of these dreamlike experiences are found in paintings like *The Wanderer* and *Paths into the Wood*.[2] In *Outline*

---

2   Nash, P. (1911) *The Wanderer*, watercolour, ink, pencil, chalk, 48.2 × 37.8 cm, Trustees of the British Museum, London; Nash, P. (1921) *Paths into the Wood*, wood engraving on paper, 12.7 × 10.2 cm, Victoria and Albert Museum, London.

he recalled this dream and how the atmosphere in the twilight of the wood influenced his work (Nash 1988 [1949]: 40). He was fascinated and completely open about recognising dominating presences and particular qualities as well as other-than-human personages within the landscapes he painted, and he felt intimately connected with them all. He saw dark places in the landscapes of his world as primeval points that bled at the margins between the worlds of the natural and the supernatural.

Several of Nash's descriptions of nature often included menace as well as wonder, obscurities and hostile places. Originally Nash experienced these places as being inexplicably dangerous. As a child he was curious but felt threatened by them. He may have been afraid of the dark places as his childhood memories suggest (Nash 1988 [1949]: 26–27). However, the manner and frequency with which he sought dark places in his art suggests interrogation and gratification rather than dread. For example, *Angel and Devil* or *The Combat* (1910), *Pyramids in the Sea* (1912) and *Nostalgic Landscape* (1922–1938) are examples of this.[3] The notion of dark places is found in the poem he wrote to accompany *Combat* where he lingers on brooding hills and dreaded places seen only in dreams. 'His imagery is informed with delicacy...poetic subtlety that does not shy away from violence and menace...' (Curiger et al. 2018: 9).

Seeing the landscape with a dark eye, as these examples clearly do, does not necessarily mean he was seeking to conjure up malevolent forces from the landscape, but rather highlight nature's inscrutability as an aspect of this world which requires our respect.

Nash was familiar with the Clumps as a boy at a time when his childhood dreams and imagination led him into fertile worlds. (Nash 1988 [1949]: 37). The reader should understand the use of the term 'imagination' as Nash used it, as 'intellectual originality, daring perception, and visionary power' (Spretnak 1999: 136) rather than Laver's emphasis on its opposition to reality (Laver 1975 [1951]: 12). On the first of August 1912, Nash wrote to Bottomley, 'I am going to Wallingford...and there hope to find some fine things.... Wonderful downs and wild woods...I have haunted them often and now I am going to try and interpret some of their secrets' (Causey 1990 [1955]: 49). At his earliest encounters with the Clumps, he knew intuitively that here was a sacred landscape with mystical, anagogic

3   Nash, P. (1910) *Angel and Devil* or *The Combat*, pen, ink and wash drawing, 35.6 × 25.8 cm, Victoria and Albert Museum, London; Nash, P. (1912) *Pyramids in the Sea*, watercolour, ink, chalk, 30.0 × 29.2 cm, The Tate Gallery, London; Nash, P. (1922–1938) *Nostalgic Landscape*, oil, 71.1 × 50.8 cm, Leicester Museum and Art Gallery, Leicester.

potential that he would return to many times. Nash reworked and explored again and again the same pictorial content. This ritualised returning to the Wittenham Clumps suggests his strong desire to participate relationally in this ancient place, or as Cardinal suggests, to 'gain deeper insight into their special magic' (Cardinal 2016 [1989]: 10). Nash's first engaged vision of it was catalytic, changing the way he thought about the larger-than-human communities at this site and in the landscape in general. Cardinal argues that Nash felt that the Clumps were 'unmistakably a landmark only to be approached in a spirit of solemnity...to its focal point of intent... what lies beneath it, a nexus of shadow which the viewer may imagine as a sanctuary' (Cardinal 2016 [1989]: 21–22).

Nash pursued an animistic response to the landscape which he felt closest to in woodlands and hedgerows. However, he was not alone in his thinking on such themes. They were also being developed in the growing liberal intellectualism reflected in the writing of E. M. Forster. In *The Longest Journey*, Forster (1907) explores the concept of other-worldly presences and the intimate relationship with landscape where he suggests that the ancient intensity of the Wiltshire countryside, its history and atmosphere might supernaturally affect or shape the course of events. Sharing a visceral sense of the visionary with Nash, he recognised the landscape as an embodied, powerful agent. It appears that both men shared a pastoral myth that associated all that is most valuable with the disappearing countryside and the sympathetic view towards paganism as well as the empathetic decline that paralleled it. Foster explored this decline in seeing anything enchanted in the world in a conversation between two of his characters discussing the medicinal properties of boar's teeth and wychelm in *Howards End* (1910). Nash reacted to this decline in his pictorial narrative, where his vision of the English landscape, and its importance to art and the English people, is clarified and conceptualised in his paintings of the Wittenham Clumps.

Within this ancient site Nash saw a deep and elusive force at work: 'Some inner design of a very subtle purpose' which he had attuned to as a child (Nash 1988 [1949]: 107). The physical and historical content of the Clumps appealed to Nash's ancestral understanding. His family had been a farming presence on the land of Buckinghamshire and Berkshire since the fifteenth century. In the eighteenth century, they had risen to greater wealth and position in landowning and the Church. By the time Nash was born, all that remained of the family material status was Langley Rectory where something of the old family ways (much enjoyed by Nash) was continued (Nash 1988 [1949]: 46–49). Anthony Bertram maintains that the peculiarly

English character of Nash's work was influenced by his Buckinghamshire background (Bertram 1955: 17). However, Cardinal feels he is drawn to the Clumps more because of the mystery surrounding them and the compositional possibilities they present. (Cardinal 2016 [1989]: 7). As I argued earlier, Nash was drawn to the landscape both by familial links and the natural qualities it offered him.

As Nash explored the nature of the landscape at the Clumps, his art began to reverberate with a sense of the sacred and his vision developed to explore the hallowed character in that landscape and his familial ties to it. He developed a pictorial language around the way he chose to perceive his ancestral landscape. These domed forms of Round Hill and Castle Hill are synonymous with his identity as a landscape painter. The landmass comprising the Wittenham Clumps is now in the guardianship of Earth Trust. The current philosophy of their work is to return the sacred hills to an engaged and active community whose relationality with the landscape and its community can cooperatively thrive (earthtrust.org.uk). This concept will be richly enhanced by engaging with Nash's artistic thrust and the way in which it situated and depicted the authority and activity that is located in this sacred landscape. In a manner now being promoted by organisations like Earth Trust, Nash explored the sacrality of the Clumps in an interactive and relational manner by engaging with a living mass of land in his unique pictorial vocabulary.

FRAMING THE VISION

Three images will be analysed as evidence of how Nash achieved an interactive engagement with these concepts in his work on the Clumps. The paintings under evaluation are *The Wood on the Hill* (1912), *Poster Design* (1913) and *Landscape of the Summer Solstice* (1943).[4] With the exception of the 1913 painting, they are devoid of human activity. It could be argued that the absence of figures gives his art a sense of melancholy and mystery. However, I maintain that human presence is omitted by Nash to desired affect: the personhood of the place, as seen and experienced by him, is present in the landscape itself.

> 4 Nash, P. (1912) *The Wood on the Hill*, pen and black ink over graphite with wash on paper, 34.3 × 33.0 cm, Ashmolean Museum, Oxford; Nash, J. & P. (1913) *Poster Design*, oil on sealing wax, in the private collection of Ms Anne Drew; Nash, P. (1943) *Landscape of the Summer Solstice*, oil, 71.8 × 91.6 cm, National Gallery of Victoria, Melbourne.

In my view, the exceptional painting that locates Nash's interactivity with the landscape is *Poster Design* (**Figure 9.2**), which he painted in collaboration with his brother John. This poster was produced by the Nash brothers for their first joint exhibition at the Dorien Leigh Gallery, London. The composition could be described as a typical multiple-registered medieval-type composition, favoured by Rossetti and others of the pre-Raphaelite movement, which in turn inspired Nash (Nash 1988 [1949]:

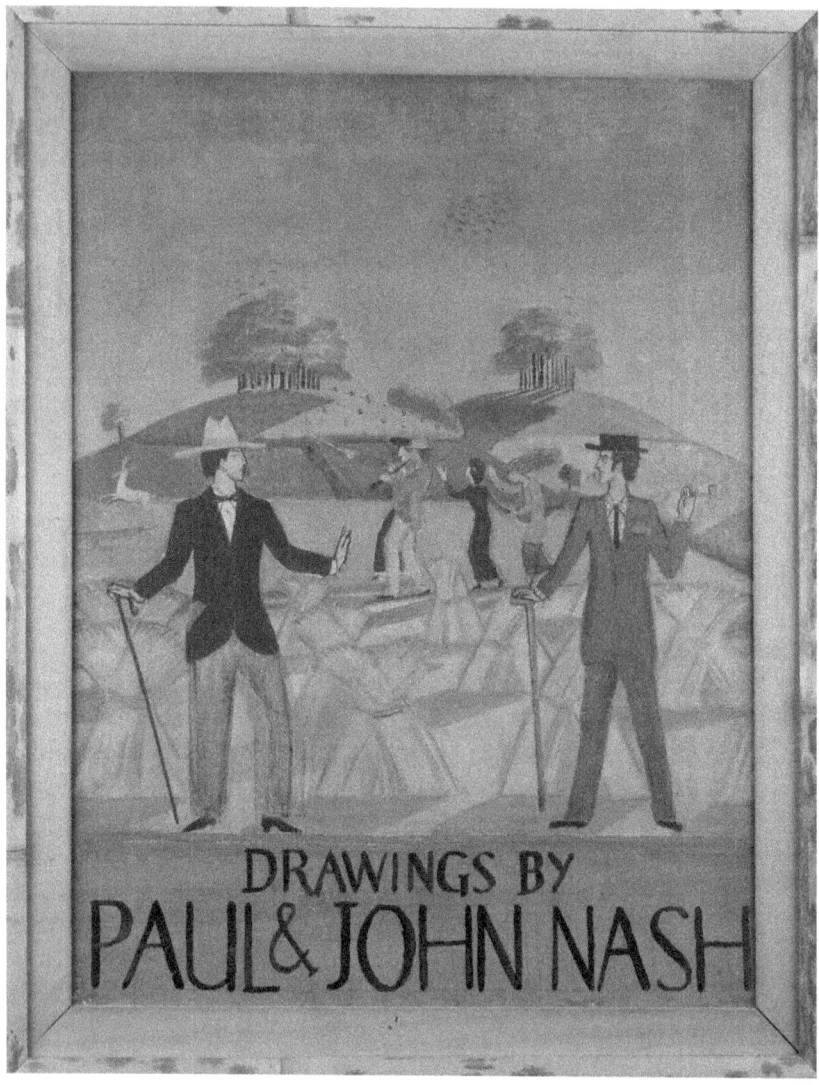

Figure 9.2 John and Paul Nash, *Poster Design*, 1913. Private collection of Ms Anne Drew.

75–76). It depicts a party of young adults at play beneath the Wittenham Clumps, which is crowned by dome-like groups of beech trees in the top register. The hills command the position of the upper background of the picture plane. In the foreground, Paul and his brother John stand in a jubilant mood, drawing the viewer into the festal scene that carries on behind them. John, on the right, dandified and pipe-smoking, directly faces Paul, who looks flamboyant in his country gentleman's attire. Standing on a lintel that separates the scene from the poster caption beneath them, they appear to have completed the last steps of a cane-enhanced dance routine. The brothers are accompanied in this dance by the three rows of embracing corn stooks positioned directly behind them. Immediately beyond the field of corn, central in the composition in the middle distance, are four frolicking adults: three women and one man. From left to right they are Rupert Lee (artist and musician and Paul's friend from the Slade) with his future wife, Rosalind Pemberton; Paul's fiancée and future wife, Margaret Odeh; and (perhaps) her friend Ruth Clark (Jenkins et al. 2010: 15). Rupert plays a flute while Rosalind, to his right, holds a cane and points their way ahead in pursuit of a white stag. The two women directly behind them, Margaret and Ruth (?), hold hands as they frisk along. The brothers have depicted the Clumps in an ecstatic romp of music and dance. Yellows, blues and reds lift the atmosphere of the frolic into a world of summer delight. Although we are not aware of how much influence his brother John exerted on this composition, since he did not return to this place in his landscape paintings, it would be a strong possibility that Paul's love of the site determined the compositional choices made.

Two very significant aspects of the work, the inclusion of the white stag and the flute, deserve special attention as they enhance Nash's vision of an engaged and relational experience of being in the landscape. The white stag appears throughout history and across cultures as a mystical symbol. The mythology can be traced through European and Asian cultures and is represented in art and legend (in Arthurian tales, pursuing the beast represents humankind's special quest to eliminate the wasteland). Nash's depiction of the stag in this work adds to the established symbolism by suggesting that once the beast is perceived and pursued, a different way of living in the landscape with interrelatedness is possible.

The inclusion of the flute in the composition echoes William Blake's and Samuel Palmer's animistic and pantheistic pastoral vision of nature (Montagu 2003: 10). From Palmer, Nash inherited the desire to explore the natural world with feelings and imagination (Vaughn 2015: 1). He also shared Palmer's desire to depict a living, vibrant landscape that connected relationally with human and other-than-human inhabitants, as well as a desire to follow his own path to otherworldliness (Wilcox 2005: 7–10; King 1987: 1). A flute-playing shepherd appears on the frontispiece of Blake's *Songs of Innocence* (1789) and in Palmer's *The Valley Thick with Corn* (1825).[5] Comparable to the white stag, the flute has its genesis within myth and legend, inextricably linked with otherworldly figures and death. For example, in Greek legends of Pan and Apollo a flute-playing contest was held before the mountain Tmolus as it was believed no one is as wise or old as the hills. During the contest, animals crept near and trees swayed in dance. The Greek myths of Undine, Syrinx and Euterpe are also associated with nature, the wild, groves, rejoicing and delight. By including the stag and flute in this composition Nash is making direct associations to the mysterious nature of the Clumps and those 'other' that dwell therein. Causey saw Nash as a Blakean conservative who valued a way of life handed down from the past, in sacred trust through many generations (Causey 2013: 34). The art of Blake drew him into emulating the chalk-like watercolours used in this depiction, which indicates the fluidity in his work and suggests the porousness of the worlds.

Referring to Nash as a scribe of the imagination situates his work within the same remit as Blake, with a firm link to the Romantics in his ontological thinking. Leonard Robinson perceives Nash as a follower of Blake and a natural Romantic (Robinson 1997: 64). In his pictorial engagement with the Clumps, Nash demonstrated his alliance to a worldview that Spretnak has termed our 'cosmological embeddedness, our dynamic participation in the sacred whole' (Spretnak 1999: 136). In pursuing his views on the importance of the visionary experience, Nash also included an element of horror in the sense of the uncanny within the landscapes that intrigued him. Nash may have been influenced by the work of Blake and Palmer but his style was 'a direct expression of his own personality' (Read 1948 [1944]: 8). Certain elements of Nash's work—his use of fantasy, imagination and the supernatural—were issues of great significance to British painters between the years 1780 and 1830 and as already noted situate his work within the Romantic imagination. Nash shared affinities with the Romantics, including prioritising a sense of emotion over reason as a tool for understanding the world. He also embraced the Romantic ideal of the artist as an inspired genius, guided by an inner vision in the process of art making. Unlike a Romantic artist such as Palmer, however, Nash argued against any

---

5   Palmer, S. (1825) *The Valley Thick with Corn*, brown ink with gum on paper, varnish, 18.2 × 27.5 cm, Ashmolean Museum, Oxford.

religious magnetism or instantaneous revelations in his work. Moreover, where many Romantics emphasised individual connections to nature and an idealised relationship to the past, Nash focused intently upon fostering a visual sense of interconnectedness. However, as already noted, although his artistic visions regarding the Wittenham Clumps were underpinned by earlier dreams and fantasies (Nash 1988 [1949]: 25–37), his adult relationship with that place was more in keeping with considerations of visual revelations.

Nash also drew inspiration from the literature and scholarship of the nineteenth century. The claim that Nash was influenced and inspired by James Frazer's *The Golden Bough* (1890), is substantiated by the 2016 catalogue *Searching for a Different Angle of Vision*, Tate Britain, which informs the reader that four books by Frazer were found in Nash's library now located in the Tate Britain archives. His library also contained a copy of Stuart Piggott's (1938) *Stukely, Avebury and the Druids*, which suggests he was very familiar with the literature surrounding the neo-pagan recovery that was taking place in the 1930s–1940s. It appears more than a possibility that he was drawn to the many anecdotes of human interaction with and theories about nature that Frazer explored. For example, Nash's *Sunflower* series from his final phase are very closely paralleled with Frazer's interest in renewal through death, an interest they shared. Frazer describes a midsummer ritual of rolling burning fire wheels down a hill to emulate the movements of the sun (Frazer 1890: chapter 62). Nash also rated highly the poetry of W. B. Yeats and in Poem 37 of *The Wind among the Reeds* (1899) he found inspiration for his art. Yeats' conception of non-physical and elemental forces surrounding and infusing humans appealed strongly to him (Nash 1988 [1949]: 84). The gold and silver of heaven's cloth, as envisioned by Yeats, is fully explored by Nash in his *Solstice* series (1942 until his death). These works reflect his participation and engagement with the emotional influence that these celestial bodies exert as they perform their dramas around the Clumps.

Nash held the opinion that his art came from what he called a 'native spring,' an Englishness that was inherent in an environment that he heard in echoes and saw in reflections (Read 1948 [1944]: 10), much deeper than the 'sympathetic imagination' Read allows him (1948 [1944]: 12). He was also finding inspiration in other materials like rotting trees and found items. Nash may not have spoken about his art as religious but Herbert Read, who knew Nash very well, stated that art for Nash was always 'a serious, even a sacred activity' (Read 1948 [1944]: 9). Nash was developing a keen interest in paganism and Druidry brought about by his visit to

Avebury in 1933. Mark Morrison claims he held 'a fascination with alternative spiritualties and epistemologies offered by occultism and esotericism' (Morrison 2017: 115). The concepts of re-enchanting the landscape that Nash was developing in his art are extensively discussed in contemporary pagan circles (Harvey 2013b: 171–186) and would have appealed to Nash.

As we have seen, Nash's childhood experience of the numinous in Kensington Gardens suggests an early acquaintance with the sense of enchantment and the otherness that reside within the landscape. 'All the senses of this growing boy, this awakening spirit, were alert, and with the passage of time their harvest was stored in the mind, to feed the imagination at need' (Read 1988 [1949]: xix). As a young boy he was fascinated by the significance of flight and light across a landscape (Nash 1988 [1949]: 26–27). In the stillness of the night a stream near his childhood home at Iver Heath became a voice that spoke to him and inspired his poetry writing. He viewed trees as personages, not the equivalent of a human form but persons in their own right. At this early stage in his life, with vitalist radar, he became aware of an essence that equated with palpable mindfulness. His earliest sightings of the Clumps appear to have caused a similar response: 'I felt their importance long before I knew their history. They eclipsed the impression of all the early landscapes I know...they were the pyramids of my small world' (Nash 1988 [1949]: 122). Cardinal appears to have caught sight of this too as he notes that despite the magnetism Nash felt for this landscape, his compositions demonstrate that they could only be approached in a mood of solemnity for what lies beneath (Cardinal 2016 [1989]: 22). Nash felt that some places defied definition, and 'they could only be indicated dumbly with a shiver or a smile' (Nash 1988 [1949]: 36). In forming a relationship with his chosen places, Nash was trying to coax these spaces into sharing some inner meaning with him. He described these sites as magical, poetic, having an aura and a sense of luminosity, awe and entrancement (1988 [1949]: 105–108). The Clumps was a space that lent itself to all of this as well as allowing Nash to visualise it in its dormant potential.

There have been numerous attempts to analyse Nash's interiorised conversations with the landscape. George Digby claimed that Nash's vision of landscape was not an intellectual one. He argued that intellect alone could not articulate what Nash was searching for. Nash explained his use of the word 'personages' referred equally to animate and inanimate objects without necessarily having any resemblance to animals or humans (Digby 1940: 111). Nash used terms like 'encounter,' 'magical places' and 'compelling Magic' when referring to the Clumps. Digby argues that Nash moved away from 'the conscious side of Man's personality, his developed civilised and thinking side' and moved towards the aniconic image (Digby 1940: 111–112). This analysis may not be suitable for all of Nash's art but it is a fair assessment of how he painted the Wittenham Clumps, even if it does not fully explain Nash's interior vision.

Causey's analysis of Nash's landscapes promotes the idea that Nash was responding to the medieval sense of *hortus conclusus*, a place of meditation (Causey 2013: 29). This also has specific connotations to the Virgin Mary, though I doubt Nash would have considered this connection other than the allusion to sacred place. Digby also felt that Nash displayed eleventh- and twelfth-century medieval characteristics in his interest in strange objects. Regarding the Wittenham Clumps, he appears to be trying to solve a riddle in much the same way we today would think about reading Anglo-Saxon art which invites careful contemplation to unravel the multilayered symbolic meanings that tell stories. Nash's pictorial responses to the Clumps provide the visual clues to help us see his vision and solve the riddle that lies within the landscape. His visual clues act as a form of meditation. As Digby and Laver see it, when Nash speaks about 'personages' and 'encounters,' he is speaking in symbols which script 'an active fantasy...which has been released by association with some external scene or image causing a harmony of utterances and a means of expression' (Digby 1940: 116; Laver 1975 [1951]: 18). Digby's analysis is thinly paralleled in Nash's paintings of the Wittenham Clumps, as in these works Nash demonstrates a familial closeness to his relational environment of mounds, sun, moon, sky, trees and flowers. Nash is very capable of unfolding a visual drama of expressions and countenances for the viewer, but, as Yorke claims, 'He had the deepest suspicion of "the psycho boys" and their attempts to probe his visions and pin them down with words' (Yorke 1988: 60). However, the 'Multi-layered gloss' that Digby and others later put on Nash's use of archetypical relics resurfaces from time to time. In the 2018 catalogue to the Arles exhibition, *Sunflower Rises*, Simon Grant suggests that Nash's mother's mental state contributed to his dark dreams and imagined 'shadow world.' He argues that Nash 'navigate[d] a pathway between the living world and that of the subconscious, the mystical and the transcendental' (Grant 2018: 75) which denies Nash's distinctive ability to know *the* world with insight and animistic relationality.

Although Digby's analysis focuses heavily on Jungian symbolism, which is not in keeping with Nash's views, he comes up with other interesting observations. In his analysis of *The Wood on the Hill*, he reads the mounds of Wittenham as representing the earth nature which gave birth to 'the race which engendered the individual' (Digby 1940: 165). According to Digby, these mounds are symbols of ascent leading upward to a divinity beyond the reach of humankind. Anne Drew shares Digby's views and sees the fences around the Clumps as emphasising their unattainability in the sense of a barrier between the sacred and the secular (perhaps in the sense of *hortus conclusus*). She argues that the birds around the beech treetops hint at the possibility of a salvation beyond, in the sense of transcendence into a holy realm (Drew 1989: 23). Drew and Digby have, in my view, misread the work. Nash was not aspiring to reach a heaven of any kind. If the pathway trope is significant, and I argue that it is, its purpose in *The Wood on the Hill* (**Figure 9.3**) is to lead us to a physical engagement with the landscape and all our relations.

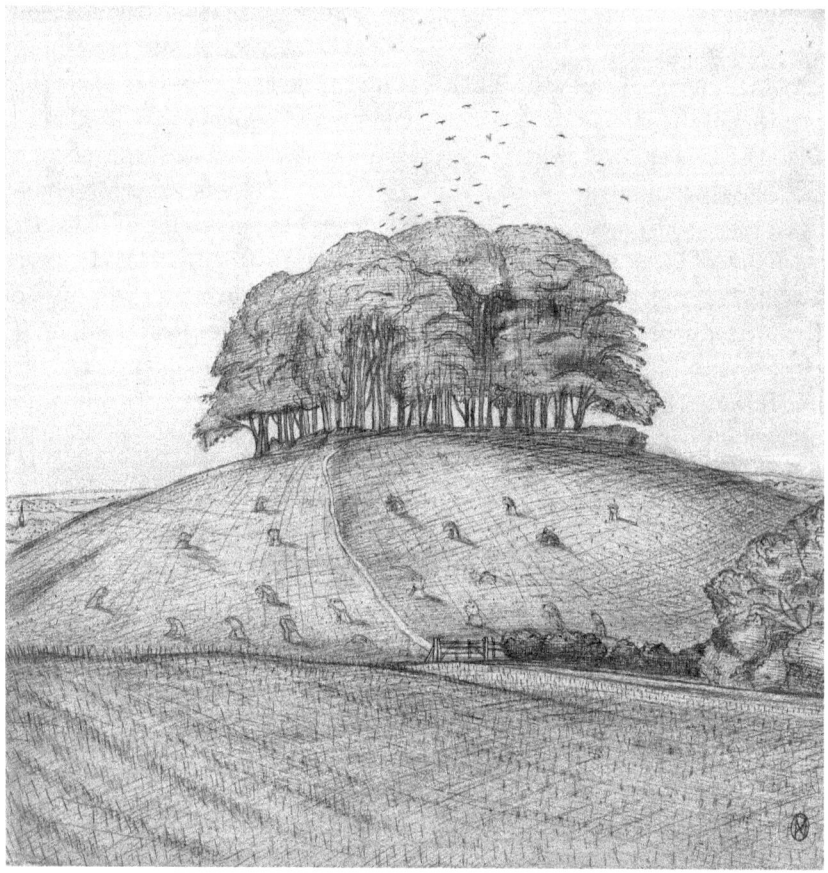

Figure 9.3 Paul Nash, *The Wood on the Hill*, 1912. © Ashmolean Museum, University of Oxford.

The Wood on the Hill is reverential, but in a more enigmatic way. It is 'captured with formal austerity and delicacy of colour...to give the sensation of a place brimming with concealed significance' (Wodehouse 2015: 228). Nash absorbed the uniqueness of the site, the numinous, the sanctity of nature and the sacredness of the landscape as it resonates with the presence of the other at the Clumps. In a letter to Bottomley (July 1945), Nash referred to his early work on the Clumps as 'In some ways the best I ever did to this day' (Letter 265, Causey 1990 [1955]: 264). Looking back on these works before his death allowed him to revisit the sense of vibrant youthfulness and energy that he depicted in the 1913 poster where he, his brother and their friends, in collaboration with their ancestors and landscape, shared great joy.

The Wood on the Hill was for Edward Ramsden the finest of Nash's drawings. He felt that Nash's 'use of economy of means...the elimination of every detail extraneous to his purpose...could hardly be bettered' (Ramsden 1948: 25). In *Outline*, Nash relates his persistent search for an angle that would convey the 'strange character' of the place (Nash 1988 [1949]: 122). He was tired and sat to eat his packed lunch and thought about the others in his family who would be eating the same lunch at that time. From this leisurely reverie on the turf beneath the Clumps he became aware of having reached his goal. This ordinary experience bonded him emotionally with his family members elsewhere within the same landscape. At that moment of familial connectedness he also felt a sensation of sacrality, knowledge that in being a part of this landscape, on this day, he had been connected to the land 'as much as my ancestors ever had' (Nash 1988 [1949]: 123). His immediate family, his predecessors and most importantly his ancient British ancestors resided in this one place. His struggles to find an absolute visual representation of the Clumps reinforced this union and his sense of his place within it.

The image of *The Wood on the Hill* draws our eyes into the symmetrically sculpted form of the wood that caps the Iron Age hill fort. Our eyes are led into the composition by the narrow line which culminates beneath the crown of trees. Very soon, we observe how Nash has deferred naturalism for 'stylised awareness' (Cardinal 2016 [1989]: 73). To the left of the wider landscape, Nash positions a tiny church spire. This could have been a compositional device to situate the Clumps in a perspectival illusion but it is more likely that he was intimating the glories of this ancient sacred place set against (as he saw it) the insignificance of an ecclesiastical edifice in the landscape. As in the 1913 poster depiction of the Clumps, the stooks of corn bow like reverent pilgrims bent in submission as they walk to the summit of sacredness above them, and to which each subsequent pilgrim will progress as part of the ritualised experience of being present in that landscape. Depicting the landscape devoid of human form, Nash enables the compelling, simple forms of pathway and corn stooks to direct the viewer's vision to the inner life of the Clumps, what Cardinal refers to as 'the calligraphic accentuation of this mystery' (2016 [1989]: 22).

Bertram argues that Nash excluded human figures because their presence was superfluous to his vision of the landscapes he painted, and maintains that Nash's uninhabited scenes create a sense of immense absence. I suggest that Nash was deliberately refraining from making humans the focus of his landscapes in order to emphasise a new way of experiencing the world as larger than human (Abrams 1997). Causey felt that for Nash 'the human face was too commonplace to record the gravity of human life' (Causey 1975 [1951]: 6). As Causey relates, Nash preferred to use inanimate objects as, rather ironically, they helped him to define human dramas (Causey 1975: 22). This technique renewed and strengthened his relationality with the landscape, and presents an opportunity for the viewer to be equally empowered by the challenge of entering the landscape. Nash's uninhabited landscapes are replete with presences, what Read referred to as 'a return to the animisms of our sacred ancestors' (1934: 246). The hill is crowned by the wood, a kind of halo encircled by birds in flight. Minute pen-scratching at the zenith of the trees gives the impression of musical notation. Nature honours nature: birds collaborate in the reverential symphonic programme of this ancient site. Their presence could be understood as a raucous veneration of nature or the sweet susurrations of whispered meditations. The manner in which he clothed this site in sacred symbols in these early visions of the Clumps indicates that Nash saw this site as potent and enigmatic.

In his final paintings, Nash returned pictorially to the Clumps in the blazing glory of sunlight and sunflower. Cardinal argues that Nash used the symbol of the sunflower to 'draw the sun close, rendering the unearthly object accessible to understanding' (Cardinal 2016 [1989]: 104). Nash may have been familiar with the Jungian readings of such images as archetypes such symbols posit but he found greater significance within the cosmic understanding of the landscapes he discovered in the writings of Frazer. Over the course of his life, he found the area evoked feelings of both the monstrous and the magical, menace and calm. He explored the mystical implication of this in his visionary landscapes. He drew on these mystical binaries, as well as the cosmic magic of the sun, in *Landscape of the Summer Solstice* (**Figure 9.4**). He saw cosmic light as supernatural and hallowed

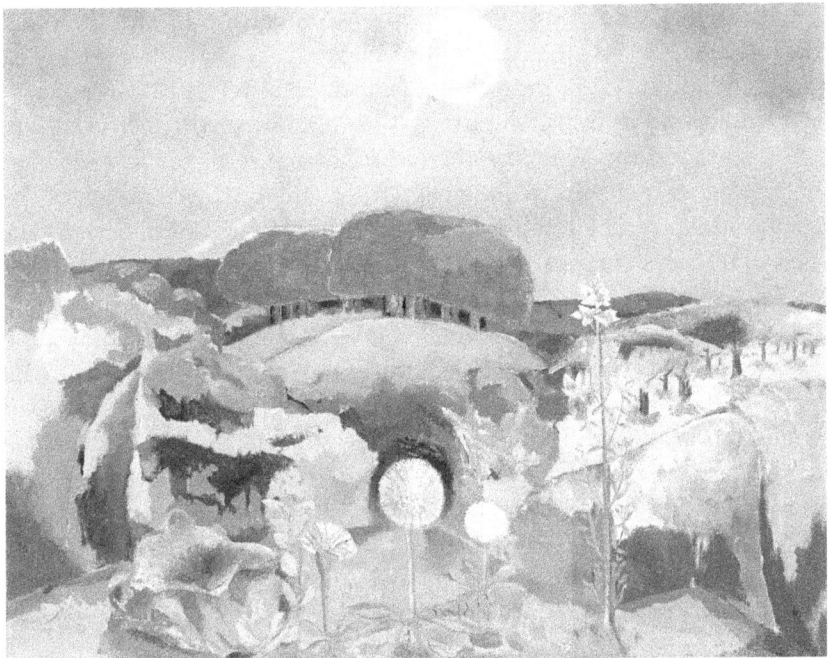

Figure 9.4 Paul Nash, *Landscape of the Summer Solstice*, 1943. National Gallery of Victoria, Melbourne.

(Nash 1988 [1949]: 35). The elements make causational appearances in these paintings. Here the cosmic and elemental love of the landscape appears.

In 1945, Nash recalled his early life and work as being complete. Looking back on them allowed him to live again that 'wonderful hour' and by returning to them he could 'finish his life' (Causey 1990 [1955]: 264). In *Landscape of the Summer Solstice*, Nash returns to the Clumps to depict their vitality and the unbounded joy he shared with that landscape. Perhaps he was returning to this landscape in the hope of locating the vision he and his young companions experienced there in the 1913 poster he created with his brother John.

Nash essentially dedicated *Landscape of the Summer Solstice* to the sun. Causey claims that Nash was greatly influenced by Francis Bain's Hindu story *The Descent of the Sun: A Cycle of Birth* (1903), which explores the sun's search for love and its achievement in forest, land and seascapes—tropes which are active in Nash's visionary landscapes (Causey 2013: 24). As his health declined he was forced to rely on field-glasses for his view of the Clumps, but, as Christopher Neve points out, he was still able to articulate the life beyond the physical despite being 'on bottled air and borrowed time' (Neve 1990: 11). His use of field-glasses caused a distortion in the viewing and renders a perspective that Cardinal refers to as 'the mystery and clarity of trans-figurative vision' (Cardinal 2016 [1989]: 115). In the foreground we enter into the distended and distorted arrangement of the flowers and shrubs of the garden, and the sunflower, at left of the composition, turning towards the sun and becoming central both to our view and Nash's purpose. The strange telescopic perspective allowed him to manipulate the surroundings and subjects in this landscape, and draws the viewer into a landscape of greater, more esoteric depth (Causey 2013: 142). As we enter Nash's image, the stem of the sunflower leads us into the frame of that vision. Cardinal argues that Nash saw the modest sunflower as 'a totem of awesome potency' (Cardinal 2016 [1989]: 104). Once again, the solitary unpeopled track to the Clumps leads us to the summit. More importantly, in this depiction we map the sunflower into the sun's rays as they cloak the Clumps in a pyramid of sumptuous glory, with the stylised treetops taking on the golden hue of the sun. Our senses are flooded with the power of the sun and its embrace of the landscape Nash loved above all others.

CONCLUSION

A liquescency of time is redolent in Nash's paintings of the Wittenham Clumps. Here the eldritch nature of the landscape demanded a focus that Nash was enchanted to depict time and time again. His vision of the Clumps allows the viewer to access the visionary pathways and arterial vigour of his artistic intellect: 'Where the ordinary mortal sees an array of facts, Paul Nash found an event' (Ramsden 1948: 31). Art-historically, Nash's depictions of the Clumps are an important contribution to the English landscape genre. Animistically, they do much more. His visual cosmology indicates an ordered plan, 'a rhythm animating the universe' (Radford 2014: 33). His vision promotes the importance of guarding and honouring our ancient, sacred past and the impact this has for the future of our connections with all our relations. At a time of distress over the stewardship of our planet, contemporary pagans and animists and all those environmentally sensitive may empathise with both Nash's vision of and personal encounters with the landscape. Nash had an affinity with the personages that he felt were inherently present within the landscape, though he sensed that both the unknown and the knowable needed to remain in order to safeguard the landscape against the sterility of pastoral niceties. In 1997, David Abrams posited a way of becoming fully human in a world full of dichotomies of culture and nature, body and mind. The fully embodied human, he suggested, was one whose every aspect of the earthly sensuous drew him or her into a relationship 'fed with curiosity and spiced with danger' (Abrams 1997: ix). From his childhood Nash was attuned to just such a relationship with his world. He negotiated relationships with his sensuous surroundings.

Nash's contribution to the English landscape painting genre is not in question. However, the importance of his vision for the future protection and honouring of our ancient landscapes has been generally overlooked. He took his landscapes beyond the physical topography to engage with the other-than-human world every time he addressed his vision towards it. Nash's religiosity is not easily encountered in a world where religious experience is often viewed as non-empirical or non-scientific. He was searching for a visual expression that laid aside what he perceived to be the baggage of institutional Anglicanism (Causey 2013: 25). In many ways, Nash saw and related to the landscape religiously, yet outside of established religious models where the natural world was secondary to humanity's concerns. His uncanny awareness of his subject subtly altered, elaborated, reinterpreted and reshaped the landscape of the Wittenham Clumps into a vision of eloquent, visual relationality that was uncommon for his time but much embraced by many today.

The challenge Nash presents to his viewer is, at its core, psychological. When we look at his representations of the Clumps, we engage in a threefold emotional engagement between Nash the artist, the landscape and ourselves: what Causey refers to as an 'emotional correspondence' (Causey 2013: 29). Having made these connections with his own experiences and the landscape, the Clumps began to shape the world for Nash. As the third party of this conversation, we the viewers become involved in the visual narratives of both the landscape and Nash's inner vision and we become aware of the connectedness that his art initiates. Nash accessed the memory that resided in the landscape of the Clumps. By doing so he stepped into the ritualised and sacralised footprint of the place. For most of his life, he was haunted by the violent nature of the material world. His war experiences had given him insight and knowledge of the world that shocked and sickened him (Read 1988 [1949]). The Clumps was one of the places where his search for a personal ontology was performed. The visual narratives written at the Clumps illuminate his search for his relational home. Nash juxtaposes the inherited ancient narrative of the Clumps with his visionary reflections to facilitate his engagement with a landscape that is animate and replete with the personages he intuitively sensed were the absolute inhabitants of this place (Causey 1988: 16).

Throughout his life, Nash challenged his viewers to see the world differently, indeed animistically. He continued to embrace what he discovered in his childhood and depicted in the 1913 poster of the Clumps. He clung to the hope that the landscape would eventually offer 'The promise of a joy utterly unreal' (Nash 1988 [1949]: 36). For Nash, the Clumps became representative of the mysterious essence he found in all landscapes. His vision of the Wittenham Clumps prompts us to look again with an animistic view to see the land relationally. Paul Nash's depictions of the Wittenham Clumps challenge contemporary society to return to the land and all our relations with respect and love. We owe it to his prophetic genius to repair the damage that our dislocation has caused.

REFERENCES

Abrams, D. (1997) *The Spell of the Sensuous*. New York: Vintage Books.
Bain, F. W. (1903) *The Descent of the Sun: A Cycle of Birth*. London: J. Parker.
Bertram, A. (1955) *Paul Nash: The Portrait of an Artist*. London: Faber & Faber.
Cardinal, R. (2016 [1989]) *The Landscape Vision of Paul Nash*. London: Reaktion Books.
Causey, A. (1975) *Paul Nash Paintings and Water Colours*. London: Tate Gallery.
Causey, A. (1975 [1951]) 'Foreword,' in Nash, M. (ed.), *Paul Nash, Fertile Image*. London: Faber & Faber, pp. 5–7.
Causey, A. (1988) 'Preface,' in Nash, P., *Outline: An Autobiography*. London: Columbus.
Causey, A. (ed.) (1990 [1955]) *Poet and Painter: Letters between Gordon Bottomley and Paul Nash*. Bristol: Redcliffe Press.
Causey, A. (2013) *Paul Nash, Landscape and the Life of Objects*. London: Lund Humphries.
Curiger, B. et al. (2018) *Sunflower Rises*. Arles: Fondation Vincent Van Gogh Arles.
Digby, G. W. (1940) *Meaning and Symbol in Three Modern Artists: Edward Munch, Henry Moore, Paul Nash*. London: Faber & Faber.
Drew, A. (1989) *Paul Nash, Places*. London: South Bank Centre.
Forster, E. M. (1907) *The Longest Journey*. Harmondsworth: Penguin.
Forster, E. M. (1910) *Howards End*. Harmondsworth: Penguin.
Frazer, J. G. (1890) *The Golden Bough*. London: Macmillan.
Grant, S. (2018) 'Into the Light,' in Curiger, B. et al., *Sunflower Rises*. Arles: Fondation Vincent Van Gogh Arles.
Hall, C. (1996) *Paul Nash, Aerial Creatures*. London: Imperial War Museum.
Harvey, G. (2005) *Animism: Respecting the Living World*. London: Hurst.
Harvey, G. (2013a) *Food, Sex and Strangers, Understanding Religion in Everyday Life*. London: Routledge. https://doi.org/10.4324/9781315729572
Harvey, G. (2013b) *The Handbook of Contemporary Animism*. London: Routledge. https://doi.org/10.4324/9781315728964
Harvey, G. (2016) 'Paganism,' in Woodhead, L., Partridge, C. and Kawanami, H. (eds.), *Religions in the Modern World*. London: Routledge, pp. 346–365.
Jenkins, D. F. et al. (2010) *Paul Nash, The Elements*. London: Scala Publications.
King, J. (1987) *Interior Landscapes: A Life of Paul Nash*. London: Weidenfeld & Nicolson.

Laver, J. (1975 [1951]) 'Introduction,' in Nash, M. (ed.), *Paul Nash, Fertile Image*. London: Faber & Faber, pp. 11–21.
Montagu, J. (2003) *Paul Nash: Modern Artist, Ancient Landscape*. London: Tate Gallery.
Morrison, M. (2017) 'The 1910s and the Great War,' in Sherry, V. (ed.), *The Cambridge History of Modernism*. Cambridge: Cambridge University Press, pp. 101–102. https://doi.org/10.1017/9781139540902.008
Nash, P. (1988 [1949]) *Outline*. London: Columbus Books.
Neve, C. (1990) *Unquiet Landscape: Places and ideas in Twentieth Century English Paintings*. London: Faber & Faber.
Radford, A. (2014) *Mary Butts and the British Neo-Romanticism: The Enchantment of Place*. London: Bloomsbury.
Ramsden, E. H. (1948) 'Wood on the Hill,' in Eates, M. (ed.), *Paul Nash, Paintings, Drawings and Illustrations*. London: Lund Humphries, pp. 22–25.
Read, H. (ed.) (1934) *Unit One*. London: Cassell and Company.
Read, H. (1948 [1944]) *Paul Nash*. Harmondsworth: Penguin Books.
Read, H. (1948) 'Paul Nash as Artist,' in M. Eates (ed.), *Paul Nash: Paintings, Drawings and Illustrations*. London: Lund Humphries, pp. 7–13.
Read, H. (1988 [1949]) 'Foreword,' in P. Nash, *Outline*. London: Columbus Books Limited, pp. xviii–xxi.
Robinson, L. (1997) *Winter Sea: The Development of an Image*. York: William Sessions Limited.
Shorter, D. D. (2016) 'Spirituality,' in Hoxie, F. E. (ed.), *The Oxford Handbook of American Indian History*. Oxford: Oxford University Press. pp. 433–450. https://doi.org/10.1093/oxfordhb/9780199858897.013.20
Sloan, K. (2017) *Places of the Mind*. London: Thames & Hudson.
Spretnak, C. (1999) *The Resurgence of the Real*. New York: Routledge.
Vaughn, W. (2015) *Samuel Palmer: Shadows on the Wall*. London: Yale University Press.
Wilcox, T. (2005). *Samuel Palmer*. London: Tate Gallery.
Wodehouse, K. (2015) 'Paul Nash 1889-1946 *The Wood on the Hill*, 1912,' in Harrison, C., et al. (eds.), *Great British Drawings*. Oxford: Ashmolean Museum, p. 228.
Yorke, M. (1988) *The Spirit of Place*. London: Constable.

Molly Kady has an MA in the Study of Religions from Winchester University where the focus of her dissertation was 'A Critical Transformation of the Jewish Soul from a Post-Patriarchal Perspective.' Her second MA in Art History from Birkbeck, London, included a study of medieval wall-paintings in English parish churches and a dissertation 'Owls, Apes and Gossips, the Othering of Jews and Women in the Fourteenth Century Misericords at Ely Cathedral.' As well as her current interest in the visionary landscape paintings of Paul Nash she is researching a project, 'The Girl with the Goat and Other Animals: The Depiction of Synagoga in Medieval Art.' Other current projects include 'Portraying the Betrayer: Depictions of Judas Iscariot in Medieval Art' and 'Menagerie in Miniature: The Animal Iconography on Bishop Fox's Chantry Chapel (1513–18).'

Chapter 10

A Hand Outstretched in Darkness: Evangelical Encounters with Art

PHILIP SALIM FRANCIS

> I grew up in a small town with almost as many churches as people. My father was the assistant pastor of an evangelical non-denominational church, so we were at church almost every day of the week. I was a good Christian boy, who loved church, sang in the choir, had crushes on Christian girls, and wanted to serve Jesus. [...] Attending Bob Jones University as an undergraduate seemed at the time like the best way to continue the intensity of my discipleship with Jesus, but in retrospect I can see how it kept me cordoned off from the rest humanity [...] You could say that the metaphorical wall between my evangelical world and the outside world was very tall, impossible to see over or to scale, but I can tell you that there were cracks in the wall. And no matter how quickly the pastors, parents and elders of our community worked to patch them up one could find small gaps if one so desired (and who didn't?). One could look through the holes, taking in that other, strange world through the eyes. One could even reach through the holes with fingers and hands, sometimes an arm would fit through all the way up to the elbow, testing out the sensations of the outside air. This is how I came across the artists whose work connected me to the outside world, who drew me into that world, and who changed the course of my life.
> —Jesse B., alumnus of Bob Jones University

Evangelicals know with certainty what scholars of religion, aesthetic theorists and neuroscientists can only gesture toward: the eye is the window to the soul—*so be careful little eyes what you see*, as the popular Christian children's song goes. This chapter explores the Herculean (often Sisyphean) efforts made by American evangelicals to avert their eyes from things unworthy of the soul. The focus is on that aspect of the visual world which evangelicals have tended to regard as the Trojan Horse of soul-polluting outsider influence, namely, the 'secular' arts. In exploring this topic, I draw primarily on my ethnographic study of over one hundred American evangelicals who left the fold through the intervention of the arts (Francis 2017). The life stories of these men and women came to me firsthand, through fieldwork, through a thousand pages of memoir written for the project, and in the hundreds of hours of conversation we have shared. All participants mark their departure from evangelicalism between the years 1980–2000 and between the ages of 20 and 30.

I came in contact with these one-time evangelicals, whom I will often refer to as 'the memoirists,' during my research on two field sites. The first site is The Oregon Extension, a semester study-away programme in the Southern Oregon Cascades, which was founded in 1975 by a small crew of renegade professors from evangelical Trinity College in Illinois. Each fall semester this small school draws between 25 and 40 students from conservative Evangelical Christian colleges, and challenges them— through fiction and poetry—to ask difficult questions of their faith. Many Oregon Extension alumni look back on their time in the programme as *the* moment in which they disavowed the 'fundamentalist side of evangelical Christianity,' as one representative alumnus puts it. The arts are often at the centre of the stories they tell.

My second field site is the Bob Jones University School of Fine Arts. This thriving art school, founded in 1947, is housed at the self-described 'fundamentalist' Christian university in Greenville, South Carolina. It has the largest faculty of any of the University's schools, and is famed for its world-class Shakespeare productions, operas, museums and galleries. For many Bob Jones students and alumni the arts go hand in hand with their faith, even if certain aesthetic experiences challenge them to revise aspects of their religious heritage. As one devout alumnus and now faculty member of the School of Fine Arts recalls: 'The arts at Bob Jones were a key part of my break with the fundamentalism of my upbringing.... Hamlet, Goethe's *Faust*, and many more…deepened and enriched my evangelical faith.' But for other Bob Jones alumni, an anguish of irreconcilability between Bob Jones-style religion and the experience of certain aesthetic masterworks sent fissures through their evangelical identity; sometimes a wrecking ball.

Jesse B., cited above, is one such alumnus of Bob Jones. In fact, Jesse's account gives the essay a focal point: the metaphorical wall which the evangelical communities of my participants constructed between themselves and the outside world, in large part to keep certain non-evangelical things—oftentimes works of art—out of sight, out of mind, out of soul.

Participants in my study almost universally bemoan the fact that in their former communities there was 'an untenably sharp line of division between Christians and non-Christians, between all things insider and all things outsider; the latter being deluded, the former purified,' as Gene E. writes in her memoir. My participants then typically go on to describe in vivid detail the ways that *the art which they beheld through the wall* helped them to undo the wall itself—'and to reengage with the fullness and messiness of the human family,' as Gene writes. Accounts such as these afford an opportunity to reflect on the wall-dismantling influence of the arts within a specific subcultural context. I conclude that these visual encounters with art-through-the-wall functioned for these one-time evangelicals as a supple medium by which to sort out and reconfigure social loyalties and disaffections—at the level of feeling, moral sensibility and desire.

FOUNDATIONS OF THE WALL: EVANGELICAL SUSPICIONS OF VISUAL ART

Space precludes a thorough accounting for the roots of evangelical suspicions of secular art, but the following snapshots give relevant context for my participants' experience. The first snapshot is of Edmund Gosse (1849–1928), the famed author and critic who, like my participants, left the Evangelical faith through the intervention of the arts. In *Father and Son: A Study of Two Temperaments* (2009 [1907]: 146), Gosse describes his departure from the faith as motivated by the observation that painting and sculpture were 'too beautiful to be so wicked as my father thought.' Of Gosse, historian David Hempton notes, 'of even more significance than theological discussions in driving Edmund to the point of separation from his father's controlling influence was his love of art and literature, a love that became the dominant passion of his adult life' (Hempton 2008: 152). Ironically, it was Edmund's father's recitation of Virgil that facilitated his son's early sense of 'the incalculable, the amazing beauty which could exist in the sound of verses' (Gosse 2009 [1907]: 143-144). And although his father would censure other artistic objects, such as works of Shakespeare, Marlowe and ancient Greek sculpture, Edmund's love for the gift of beauty could neither be undone nor reconciled with an evangelical faith: 'the magic of [beauty] took hold of my heart for ever' (Gosse 2009 [1907]: 143-144).

Gosse demonstrates just how deep evangelical suspicions of art run in the tradition and how irresistible is art's influence when viewed through the wall of prohibition. Like the evangelical tradition as a whole, Gosse's father embodies long-standing Christian ambivalences about pleasure, beauty and the visual. For Evangelicals, these ambivalences were shaped into convictions by way of the lingering influence of certain Calvinist strands of its Protestant Reformation heritage. Famously, reformers such as Calvin and Zwingli railed against the sensual visuality and idolatrous level of Catholic devotion to painting and statuary. These polemics, in turn, find their way into the heart of Gosse's father and into the evangelical bloodstream by way of proto-evangelicals George Whitfield and others in the formative eighteenth and nineteenth centuries. In the early twentieth century, not long after Gosse penned *Father and Son*, nascent evangelicalism was further shaped by the cross currents of the 'fundamentalist-modernist' controversies. These debates, though not centred on theological aesthetics, cemented the evangelical self-understanding as an embattled community with a rearguard against all things modern: modern culture, modern art and most of all modern religion.[1]

A second snapshot, again of a father and son. If we fast-forward through the twentieth century—the 'Evangelical century' in America—to the 1970s, which is the birth decade of the majority of my participants, we find that the evangelical suspicion of art remains palpable and often critiqued. Sometimes the critique arises from within the ranks, a reminder that evangelicalism is not and never has been monolithic. That a highly influential evangelical thinker such as Francis Schaeffer, who in the 1970s had his finger on the pulse of the evangelical world, would open his 1973 book in defence of art with the following rhetorical questions is indication of the low esteem in which many evangelicals held the arts in the era in which my participants were raised: 'Is art—especially the fine arts of painting and music—simply a way to bring in worldliness through the back door? [...] Shouldn't a Christian focus his gaze steadily on "religious things" alone and forget about art and culture?' (Shaeffer 2006 [1973]: 1). Shaeffer knows that his evangelical readership will tend to assume that art

---

1 For the context of these debates and their influence on American religion see: Marsden (2006); Taves (1999); Schmidt (2005); Schmidt (2008). My understanding of the fundamentalist and evangelical approaches to the arts is also influenced by Doreen M. Rosman's survey (1984) of evangelical approaches to the theatre, novel-reading, the fine arts and other aspects of culture, as well as Francis Shaeffer's influential booklet *Art and the Bible* (1973) and thoughtful responses to Shaeffer by Daniel Siedell (2008) and William Dyrness (2001). For evangelical and fundamentalist approaches to culture in general and the life of the mind in particular, see Noll (1994).

is at best a distraction from the things of God, and at worst a corrupting, 'worldly' influence.

Shaeffer's son, Franky Shaeffer, elaborated in a tone far more biting than his father's, but no less revealing as an insider account: 'The arts, cultural endeavors, enjoyment of beauty, enjoyment of creativity...these creative gifts have in our century and day and age been relegated to the bottom drawer of [evangelical] Christian consciousness, despised outright as unspiritual or unchristian' (Shaeffer 1981: 16). Given this unequivocal tone, it will come as no surprise that Franky, like Gosse, left the evangelical fold of his father in pursuit of the beauty of the arts, which he comes to find in Eastern Orthodox iconography and his own artistic pursuits. Evangelical approaches to art have changed, in some quarters, over the last thirty-five years.[2] But the Shaeffers' critiques continue to resonate through the accounts of my participants. So then, when my participants refer to the wall between the evangelical world and the artwork of the outsider, it is important to recognise that its foundation is centuries old and it has been reinforced since their earliest memories by way of very clear distinctions between 'good' and 'bad' kinds of 'aesthetic' experience. Bad aesthetic experiences were Catholic, secular and sensual. The good were Jesus-centred, didactic and rare.

As my participant Annie C. recalls in her memoir, 'I grew up in a compartmentalised world. Everything, especially music and art, was separated into categories of Christian and secular.' Bryan H.'s memoir puts it this way: 'Directly and indirectly, I was taught that Satan lurked in the outside world, and that the door to that world was *secularist* material. If the philosophy, music, art, literature, or poetry wasn't in the Bible, or it didn't have that spin on it...it was banished as faulty or sinful.' Numerous participants recall being asked to destroy all of their secular and non-evangelical art upon conversion to the faith. I can still recall 'the smell of burning vinyl on the day I was born again,' recalls participant Jakob Z. memorably. 'Even just the possibility that we might look upon the album covers was reason enough to toss them in the fire. Eliminating the sight of these things was always presented as a first line of defence against falling to temptation.'

---

2 In addition to the Shaeffers, the following organisations and publications have been influential: the journal *Image!*, founded by writer Gregory Wolfe in 1989 as a site of reflection on 'Art, Faith, Mystery'; and the International Arts Movement (IAM), founded by visual artist and evangelical Christian, Makoto Fujimura in 1992.

My participants tell me that in their former communities only a small band of individuals was safe from the outsider label. Even the majority of other, self-proclaimed Christians were categorised as outsiders. This categorisation could be applied to large, self-describing Christian institutions: 'I remember one particular lesson on why the Catholic Church was a cult of idol worshippers and the Pope was the Anti-Christ,' recalls Holly S. And it could be applied with equal fervour to many small cultural moments: 'I worked at the radio station at [evangelical College in North East],' says Violet W., 'and remember hating not being able to play certain music even by explicitly [Protestant] *Christian* bands if it wasn't on *Word Music*'s label [a conservative Christian music label]. That was how "Christian Rock" was narrowly defined by the college.'

If certain Protestant Christian artists were out of bounds, then all the more were the obviously 'secular.' Several memoirists in this study recall that after their conversion, or the conversion of their parents, to these particular forms of Christianity they were instructed to destroy all of their 'non-Christian' art and music. Cameron S. writes, 'It was in the little things; like I wasn't allowed to listen to non-Christian music and I remember it was scandalous to my mom when I watched *Titanic* (my senior year in high school) because it condoned pre-marital sex!' Participant Mary S., who attended Bob Jones University adds, '[O]ur music had to be checked by the [Bob Jones] administration (most genres were excluded if "sensual" electric guitars and "sexual" drumbeats were present) and so forth.' As in these accounts, the tight controls on music and art rivalled the regulation of sexuality, and frequently the two were interrelated. While conducting fieldwork at Bob Jones School, I was invited by Jay Bopp, the chair of the Division of Art and Design, to visit a studio art class in progress: eight or so students stood at easels, working on various still-lifes—fruits, vegetables, flowers, *no* nudes. 'We make sure that students get a foundation in classical realism before they do anything abstract,' Jay informed me. 'Do you use nude models?' I asked. 'No,' he replied, unflustered. 'We think it is too much of an occasion for temptation for undergraduates.'

The language of corruptions, pollutants and impurities is common in these characterisations of art from the outside world. Participant Sandy W. recounts the day her parents discovered that she had visited the Museum of Fine Arts in Boston. 'They found the ticket stub, sat me down, and lectured me on the dangers of spending time in the company of artists who would pervert our understanding of God's vision for the world. They prayed over me at the end of the conversation. I don't remember the exact words but it had the quality of an exorcism, like they were casting out the influence of evil artists that had entered my being when I looked at their art.' Participant James S. recalls a time when the headmaster of his Christian high school publicly shamed a group of students into tearing up and throwing away their tickets to a Pearl Jam concert (and in the 1990s Pearl Jam tickets had great cultural significance). 'He told us that even if we sold the tickets to someone else we would be guilty of corrupting that person through our moral failure,' James recalls.

Participant Todd B. includes the following recollection in his memoir:

> While entrenched in fundamentalism I found it difficult to enjoy any art that was even slightly outside the 'safety zone of approval'.... This narrow, fear-based perspective robbed me of innumerable opportunities to appreciate art. When my wife and I were in the first stages of 'disentanglement' [from fundamentalism] my mother (who remains entrenched in fundamentalism) was visiting our home. I was playing with our six-year-old son—just playing, singing, and enjoying one another. I specifically remember that we were singing the Willie Nelson cover of Arlo Guthrie's 'City of New Orleans'. My mother was disturbed by this and told me, 'You do know that you are teaching him ROCK MUSIC don't you?' Her implication was that my positive interaction with my son was going to somehow set him on a pathway of moral degradation. I was angered by her unwillingness to see the positive relationship that was developing between her son and grandson.

The road to perdition, in the mind of Todd's mother, was paved with outsiders' art. The distinction between insider and outsider was so vivid in her mind, suggests Todd, that the positive relationship between her son and grandson was obscured. Indeed, the practice of dividing up the world between insiders and outsiders was so prevalent in these communities that the attempt to think and act beyond and without this conceptual binary proved exceptionally difficult for many of the participants in this study—even after leaving conservative church communities far behind.

Todd recalls,

> The transition away from my old way of thinking was sometimes traumatic. While in grade school, high school, and college I always had a Christian teacher, professor, etc. who was responsible for 'approving' music and movies that were suitable for Christian life. When I began disentangling from that system of thinking I often found myself feeling as if I needed someone's approval for decisions that most people would make on their own.

As accounts such as these make legible, most of my participants were strongly discouraged, through a range of teachings and practices, from consorting with outsiders, and frequently it was the outsiders' works of art that were understood to give most potent expression to deluded states and sinful desires. And so the intention to keep the influence of outsiders at bay, to keep *their* desires from before the eyes, was closely allied with a prohibition against outside artistic forms. What better way to prevent visual encounter than to build a psychological or spiritual wall?

The above discussion should not obscure the fact that the evangelical commitment to keeping secular art out of sight arises, at least in part, from a deep conviction about the great power of art to influence not only our moral character but our *eternal destiny*. Formation in evangelicalism thus leaves my participants uniquely sensitised to the powerful effects of art on their spiritual journey, on earth as well as in heaven. The fact that the border between evangelical insiders and outsiders were often drawn along aesthetic lines granted the arts more power still. With just this schematic sense of evangelical approaches to the secular and non-evangelical arts in place, my reader can likely begin to imagine the ways art might come to facilitate the process by which my participants literally *see and feel* their way out of evangelicalism and into other social units.[3]

FISSURES IN THE WALL: INABILITY TO VILIFY BEAUTY

It turns out that the art of non-evangelicals is not so easily banished, even with high walls and vigilant guards. Recall that in Jesse's account, as in Gene's and Bryan's, the artwork of the outsider seeps through thick walls and destabilises carefully constructed lines of demarcation, like those between insider and outsider, evangelical and other. Take the account of Jakob Z., cited above, who writes, 'There never would have been an undoing of my conservative Evangelical worldview without my encounter with the transcendent work of Mark Rothko on that rainy afternoon in London's Tate Modern. I sat there for five hours and everything came undone.' London, rain and Rothko: each was foreign to the missionary encampment on the Navajo reservation where Jakob grew up, in the 1980s. Back then he seized every opportunity to share the gospel with his Native American friends, even as they played endless games of cowboys and Indians in the deserts of Arizona: 'the Navajo kids always wanted to be the cowboys, because the cowboys always win, they said.' Into his early twenties, Ivis

---

3 'Literally feel' is a phrase used by David Morgan in *The Embodied Eye: Religious Visual Culture and the Social Life of Feeling* (2012: 146).

assumed that he would follow in the footsteps of his Pentecostal parents, attend Bible school, and enter into full-time ministry. He nearly did. But then, on a trip to the UK, Jakob experienced an irresistible urge to explore the art museums of London, though he knew his family and evangelical community would frown on such exploration. He found his way to the Tate Modern:

> Wandering through its galleries, I came into a room that was dimly lit. The space had the feel of a small chapel. There were benches in the middle of the space, one for each wall. The space was quiet. There were a few people seated on the benches who seemed completely transfixed by the paintings in the space. As I looked around, I realized all the paintings in the space were similar enough to have been created by the same artist and seemed to envelop the gallery; they stretched from floor to ceiling and butted up against one another. [...] I too soon became transfixed, sat on one of the benches and stared at the paintings for hours, finding both strangeness and comfort in their form. [...] It was seemingly otherworldly. Upon leaving the gallery, I found out that the painter was Mark Rothko, and I told myself I wanted to do for someone else what he had done for me.[4]

Elsewhere in his memoir Jakob declares, 'If it weren't for the arts—Rothko, Bob Dylan, Hemingway, Kerouac, to name a few—I am not sure there would have been an unsettling of my evangelical certainties. Aesthetic experiences burst the Evangelical Christian bubble that was my world.' Jakob's account suggests that art had the unique ability to penetrate the very wall erected to keep it out. In one sense, the accounts of Jakob and my other participants can be read as a vindication of the worst fears of evangelical leaders: viewing the art of outsiders made them outsiders themselves.

Participant Joe S. recounts a similar scenario:

> In the church where I grew up, there was good music and Devil's music. And I really believed this—with my head. But my heart could not be kept from music of all kinds. I remember hearing U2's *The Joshua Tree* album at my babysitter's house. Those songs lit up places in my mind and imagination that I didn't know existed. It was like nothing else. I was overwhelmed by the sheer beauty of 'Where the Streets Have No Name.' There were many times when I listened to 'secular' music and felt guilty afterwards: Am I desensitising myself to the influence of evil? Is my babysitter a 'false' Christian?

---

4 On aesthetico-religious experiences evoked by Rothko, see: Elkins (2005) and Rosen (2016).

But during the actual experience of something like 'Where the Streets Have No Name,' there was no thought that this could be from the Devil. It was too beautiful. I was overwhelmed.

Like Edmund Gosse, Jakob and Joe find it exceptionally difficult to categorise the work of art as 'of the evil one,' even when all the authority figures in their lives, and indeed their formation in an insiders-versus-outsiders worldview, have convinced them—'in their head'—that this is the case. There is something in beauty and art, as they pass through the blockade to the outside world, that calls into question the moral valuation of a division between insider and outsider, that overwhelms and transgresses the boundaries.

A rather striking revelation is implicit in these accounts, and in the stories of a number of the memoirists in my study. They found themselves able to maintain the wall between 'all things insider' and 'all things outsider' when it came to the consideration of beliefs, moral codes *and* other people. But they found it impossible to maintain this division when it came to beauty and art. It was easier, at least initially, they suggest, to characterise other ('outsider') human beings as evil than it was to characterise 'the gift of beauty' as being of the evil one. What begins as an inability to characterise artworks as evil becomes a refusal to maintain the division between insiders and outsiders in other regards as well. For Joe, Jakob and the others, once art had created a crack in the wall between insiders and outsiders, there was frequently the desire—slow-burning though it sometimes was—to tear down the wall completely.

Participant Eliza F.'s memoir suggests something similar:

From my earliest memories, I had crayons, coloured pencils, paintbrushes and markers always in my hands. I could spend hours creating pictures of the world around me and the world within me. Like any parents would, my super duper evangelical parents saw no harm in this when I was a kid. Most of my pictures were about church stuff anyways. [...] But I distinctly remember that they grew more and more anxious about my love of creating visual images as I grew older, especially as I wanted to take art classes and explore museums, which they forbade. My get around was to go to the library and take down those heavy, glossy books full of great works of art. I'd find hidden parts of the library to just sit and soak in the visual genius of those works through my little eyes. Inevitably, when I was 17 years old my hyper vigilant mother caught me looking at these books (specifically a book of Matisse). She shamed me, in what I now realise were sexualised terms: 'You are adulterating the lily white soul that Jesus gave you,' she said. 'You are corrupting yourself with these secular images. We don't see the world like they do.' Of course this cut deep, and honestly looking back now as a 35-year-old woman, I cannot believe that I responded the way I did. I was quiet as I put the books back on the shelf. And I am sure that my mother thought I had taken the rebuke to heart. But as it cut deep a fissure opened up. Far from taking her word as sacred writ, I was having a revelation about her fallibility. I realised in some unshakable way that if she could be so wrong about these beautiful images then she could be wrong about other things as well. She could be wrong about Jesus, about the Bible, about the whole truth of our evangelical brand of Christianity. My father could be wrong too. And our pastor [...]. I resolved to side with the makers of beautiful things. It was on that day that I became an artist. But ah, the guilt that still plagued me.

Later in her memoir, Eliza recalls an overwhelming sense of solidarity with the title character in Chaim Potok's novel, *My Name is Asher Lev*, which she read in her early twenties. Young Asher grows up in a Hasidic community in which his preternatural ability to create drawings and paintings is frowned upon by his parents, his teachers and his rabbi. He is told that in exercising the gift he is acting like the *Goyim*—the outsiders. He is told that his gift is given to him by the evil One, the ugly One, working through the influence of outsiders. Asher is disturbed by these accusations. He takes them seriously. He attempts to put down the pencil and the brush but cannot. Yet, as with Eliza, something in the logic of the admonitions coming down to him from these authority figures does not add up: 'It was horrifying to think my gift [of drawing and painting] may have been given to me by the source of evil and ugliness [as the rabbi claimed]. How can evil and ugliness make a gift of beauty? I lay in my bed and thought a long time about what was wanted from me,' recalls Asher (Potok 1972: 119).

The very question that troubled Asher Lev and Edmund Gosse—of evil's relationship to the creative arts—is at play for Eliza. As with Gosse, Lev, Joe and Jakob, strikingly, Eliza's loyalty remained with beauty and the arts rather than the deep-seated controlling influences of family and religion. It was through her refusal or inability to categorise art as good or evil, insider or outsider, that she began to question the adequacy of these divisions in other regards. If she could not trust her mother or her church community to make decisions about visual art, then perhaps they were suspect in other ways as well. 'In what other ways might they be wrong about the outside world.' From this line of thought came a new mindset for Eliza, one of 'self-reliance,' she says, the realisation that she could 'choose for herself.' Quite directly, then, it was her love for visual art that cast a shadow of suspicion over her church community and across the divide between insiders and outsiders. Aesthetic experience, mediated by the wall, generated that small crack in the foundation of the structure that sent splintery fingers through the whole, and eventually brought it down.

THE WALL COMES DOWN: ART AND THE DESIRES OF OTHERS

Participant Barry H. tells me that his grandfather and his father were evangelical preachers, and his mother a faith healer. 'You could say I inherited an unshakeable fundamentalist Christian mindset from my family.' This unshakable faith was maintained, at least in part, 'by minimising contact with non-believers,' recalls Barry, except for purposes of evangelising—and except in the form of celluloid. In his late teens and early twenties, Barry became obsessed with film, and began working his way through various *Top 100 Movies of All Time* lists. A deep sense of kinship with the actors, directors and the films themselves began to take root in Barry's consciousness. This sense culminated in the summer of 1996, when in a musty basement in suburban Memphis, Tennessee, twenty-five-year-old Barry encountered the films of David Lynch, Krzysztof Kieslowski and Ingmar Bergman. 'These films,' he says, 'made me tremble with recognition that the full range of human needs, wants, fears and longings were as intimately woven into my being as they were into anyone else's—Christian or non-Christian. I could no longer deny it. And I didn't want to.' The stony wall of division between himself and all non-evangelicals 'came tumbling down.'

Barry tells me that this recognition,

> took several months to sink in, as the experiences of the films did work on me. The characters from [Lynch's] *Blue Velvet*, [Kieslowski's] *The Colors Trilogy* and [Bergman's] *Winter Light* got right into my unconscious. I still have dreams where I have brief conversations with Pastor Tomas in *Winter Light*. I can never remember anything we say to each other but the general feeling is of a mutual forgiveness, like 'we didn't know any better; it's how we were raised, let's be forgiving of ourselves.' Actually lots of the characters from these films still show up in my dreams and stray thoughts and in my photography. These films changed the way I think about [photography] too. I want to communicate to the people who see my work what these films communicated to me, which is basically the human condition—the human soup that we are all soaked through with. We just are not that different when you take away the externals—we all want the same good and bad things. But we build up massive systems of belief to try to deny this. I'm done with that.

It was this recognition—this unsettling of the wall between insiders and outsiders *at the level of aesthetics and desire*—that prompted Barry to break with the church community of his upbringing: 'After I had this epiphany, whenever I would go to church, the way that they would isolate themselves from the outside world, and speak in different terms about those outside of the church sickened me. At first, I would argue with them. Pretty soon, I couldn't take it anymore.'

The accounts of my participants, like Barry, make the case again and again. The desires of outsiders, they tell us, were viewed as repulsive and corrupting agents in their evangelical communities; and the arts were viewed as conduits of such corruption. Yet, many of these same participants, like Barry, hold that the arts, under these wall-mediated circumstances, helped them to undo the repulsion they felt toward the desires of others and in this way helped them to undo the divide between insider and outsider. What constellation of context and effect must be in place to cause a moviegoer like Barry to tremble 'with recognition that the full range of human needs, wants, fears and longings were as intimately woven into my being as they were into anyone else's'? At some fundamental level, this recognition disrupts Barry's performance of the insider's identity, an identity premised upon its distinctiveness from the outsider whose alien desires threaten and repulse.

Given that a great many leading thinkers—of persuasions as diverse as Henry Thoreau and Sigmund Freud—have fallen sway to the idea that art entails the power to break down the barriers between insiders and outsiders, perhaps it is unsurprising that so many of my participants employ a similar language to describe the role of the arts in their break with evangelicalism. They may simply be channelling that pervasive romantic belief which lies at the heart of Thoreau's epigram: *'when I hear music...I see no foe'* (Thoreau 2009: 621). That art possesses the ability to transcend the boundaries that cordon us off from fellow human beings—boundaries cultural, racial, creedal and linguistic—is almost an article of faith among certain heirs of romanticism, especially among modern artists and theorists of the aesthetic. In aesthetic experience, the claim goes, the us-versus-them mentality dissolves into a pool of deeper unities. John Dewey summarises his own version of this belief succinctly:

> [Artistic] expression strikes below the barriers that separate human beings from one another. Since art is the most universal form of language, since it is constituted, even apart from literature, by the common qualities of the public world, it is the most universal and freest form of communication.... The

sense of communion generated by a work of art may take on a definitively religious quality.... Art is the extension of the power of rites and ceremonies to unite men through a shared celebration, to all incidents and scenes of life.... That art weds man and nature is a familiar fact. Art also renders men aware of their union with one another in origin and destiny. (Dewey 2005: 271)

Like so many aesthetic theorists before and after him, Dewey's purported secularism and disciplined anti-utopianism give way to effusions about the salvific efficacy of aesthetic experience—in explicitly religious terms.

If Thoreau's or Dewey's optimism sounds inflated on this point, perhaps Sigmund Freud's highly *uncharacteristic* optimism better demonstrates the pervasiveness of the idea—and how difficult it is to shake:

On learning of the [the fantasies of the other] we are repelled by them or at best feel cool towards them. However, when a creative writer presents his plays to us [or his personal fantasies] we experience a great pleasure, and one which probably arises from the confluence of many sources. How the writer accomplishes this is his innermost secret; the essential *ars poetica* lies in the technique of overcoming the feeling of repulsion in us which is undoubtedly connected to the barriers that rise between each single ego and the others. (Freud 2003: 33)

After being immersed in the accounts of my participants like Barry, John Dewey's claim that art is a 'universal form of communication,' striking below the barriers that 'separate human beings from one another,' sounds less starry-eyed. In these accounts, aesthetic experiences do function, in a sense, as means of communication that override the barriers between insider and outsider. In their accounts, it is the artist who communicates her hopes and desires, her sense of the messiness of life, indeed, her own humanity in maximally creative and compelling ways. But, of course, there is no guarantee that such communication, no matter how compelling, will render insiders and outsiders 'aware of their union with one another in origin and destiny,' as Dewey opines. So much depends on context and reception.

Immersion in the accounts of my participants leads me to believe that it is more adequate to say that the arts create *unpredictable* 'forms of sympathy, empathy, antipathy, and apathy—feeling with, feeling into or as, feeling against or other than,' as David Morgan says of visual images (2012: 147). That is, particular artworks, under certain conditions, in specific contexts, may generate an experience of the desirability of larger communities of agreement, and even exert a low-flying pressure toward such communion. And in the accounts of certain of my participants, it is undeniably the case that art created small, unforeseeable pockets of commonality between themselves and certain outsiders, *sui generis* communities gathered spontaneously around common objects of desire, the desire for which remained always just beyond their ability to articulate within a set of familiar concepts and categories (Nehamas 2010: 81).[5]

In this sense, what contemporary philosopher Alexander Nehamas says of beauty applies to a broader set of aesthetic experiences: 'far from being selfish or solipsistic, the desire beauty provokes is essentially social: it literally does create a new society, for it needs to be communicated to others and pursued in their company' (2010: 77). If the arts do not necessarily 'unite *all* people' under one banner, as Dewey would have it, they may at least unite individuals with other individuals with whom they might not otherwise have been united. That is to say, art may generate communion between people in a manner that cuts across their other forms of communal identity—by resisting conceptualisation and comparison, by engendering empathy, by awakening desires—and so undercut the wall between insider-outsider. Indeed, in the accounts gathered in these pages, there is repeated reference to a *felt-sense* of communion (with artists and outsiders), which is engendered through seeing their work through the wall. This felt-sense of communion, my memoirists say, cuts unpredictably across other forms of communal identity, and so destabilises their sharp dividing lines between insiders and outsiders. To find themselves suddenly sharing common ground, indeed common aesthetic objects of desire, with persons previously branded as 'outsiders,' often occasioned a thoroughgoing revision of their evangelical identity, exactly because such a great extent of that identity was premised on maintaining a clear wall of delineation between insiders and outsiders.

Running through the stories of my participants is the common experience of encountering the unexpected through art and beauty. In one way or another, each of my memoirists discovered something unforeseen about

---

5   Nehamas follows Ted Cohen (see Cohen 1988: 12) and David Carrier. Carrier argues that 'The values of morality bind us to one another. They move us to expand the circle of our concern as widely as we possibly can and, for that reason, both exploit and generate similarities among us. Aesthetic values have a narrower domain. They direct us to smaller and more special groups, which stand out against the rest of the world and within which it is possible for us, too, to stand out' (Carrier 2003: 86).

the outsider, or the outside world, in and through aesthetic experience as mediated by the wall. Elaine Scarry's description of 'beauty's welcome' adds a more personalised interpretive layer to the unexpectedness contained in these experiences, especially as they transpire *through the wall*.

> Not Homer alone but Plato, Aquinas, Plotinus, Pseudo-Dionysius, Dante, and many others repeatedly describe beauty as a 'greeting'. At the moment one comes into the presence of something beautiful, it greets you. It lifts away the neutral background as though coming forward to welcome you…it is as though the welcoming thing entered into, and consented to, you being in its midst. Your arrival seems contractual, not just something you want, but something the world you are now joining wants. (Scarry 2001: 25–26)

Consider what a strange mix of emotions someone like Jesse, who provided the metaphor of the wall at the outset of this chapter, must have felt upon the experience of beauty's welcome. An innocent onlooker, he peers sheepishly out through a small gap in that tall metal fence that runs between his world and that of the outsiders. Expecting to encounter who knows what kind of strange thing, his gaze fastens upon an object that 'lifts away from the neutral background as though coming forward to welcome [him].' Though his gaze is unlawful, he is welcomed warmly. Though apparently on the other side of a great wall, beauty calls out in greeting: Come friend, there is no fence between us. Good fences do not make good neighbours.

BIBLIOGRAPHY

Carrier, David. (2003) *Writing about Visual Art*. New York: Allworth Press.
Cohen, Ted. (1988) 'The Very Idea of Art,' *NCECA Journal*, 9, 12–17.
Dewey, John. (2005) *Art as Experience*. New York: TarcherPerigee.
Dyrness, William. (2001) *Visual Faith: Art, Theology, and Worship in Dialogue*. Grand Rapids, MI: Baker Academic.
Elkins, James. (2005) *Pictures and Tears: A History of People Who Have Cried in Front of Paintings*. New York: Routledge. https://doi.org/10.4324/9780203990322
Francis, Philip Salim (2017). *When Art Disrupts Religion: Aesthetic Experience and the Evangelical Mind*. New York: Oxford University Press. https://doi.org/10.1093/acprof:oso/9780190279769.001.0001
Freud, Sigmund. (2003) 'The Creative Writer and Daydreaming,' in *The Uncanny*. London, Penguin.
Gosse, Edmund. (2009 [1907]) *Father and Son: A Study of Two Temperaments*. New York: Oxford University Press.

Hempton, David. (2008) *Evangelical Disenchantment: Nine Portraits of Faith and Doubt*. New Haven, CT: Yale University Press.
Marsden, George. (2006) *Fundamentalism and American Culture*, second edition. Oxford: Oxford University Press.
Meyer, Brigit. (2008) 'Powerful Pictures: Popular Christian Aesthetics in Southern Ghana,' *Journal of the American Academy of Religion*, 76(1), 82–110.
https://doi.org/10.1093/jaarel/lfm092
Morgan, David. (1996) *Icons of American Protestantism: The Art of Warner Sallman*. New Haven, CT: Yale University Press.
Morgan, David. (1998) *Visual Piety: A History and Theory of Popular Religious Images*. Berkeley, CA: University of California Press.
Morgan, David. (1999) *Protestants and Pictures: Religion, Visual Culture, and the Age of American Mass Production*. Oxford: Oxford University Press.
Morgan, David. (2003) 'Aesthetics,' in Hillerbrand, Hans (ed.), *The Encyclopedia of Protestantism*, 4 vols. New York: Routledge, vol. 1, pp. 7–8.
Morgan, David. (2012) *The Embodied Eye: Religious Visual Culture and the Social Life of Feeling*. Berkeley, CA: University of California Press.
https://doi.org/10.1525/california/9780520272224.001.0001
Nehamas, Alexander. (2010) *Only A Promise of Happiness*. Princeton, NJ: Princeton University Press
Noll, Mark. (1994) *The Scandal of the Evangelical Mind*. Grand Rapids, MI: Eerdmans.
Potok, Chaim. (1972) *My Name is Asher Lev.* New York: Knopf.
Rosen, Aaron (ed.). (2016) *Religion and Art in the Heart of Modern Manhattan: St. Peter's Church and the Louise Nevelson Chapel*. New York: Routledge.
https://doi.org/10.4324/9781315604725
Rosman, Doreen M. (1984) *Evangelicals and Culture*. London: Croom Helm.
Scarry, Elaine. (2001) *On Beauty and Being Just*. Princeton, NJ: Princeton University Press.
Schmidt, Leigh. (2005) *Restless Souls: The Making of American Spirituality from Emerson to Oprah*. New York: Harper Collins.
Schmidt, Leigh. (2008) *Unsettled Minds: Psychology and the American Search for Spiritual Assurance 1830-1940*. Berkeley, CA: University of California.
Shaeffer, Francis. (2006 [1973]) *Art and the Bible*. Downers Grove, IL: InterVarsity Press.
Shaeffer, Franky. (1981) *Addicted to Mediocrity: 20th Century Christians and the Arts*. Wheaton, IL: Crossway Books.
Siedell, Daniel. (2008) *God in the Gallery: A Christian Embrace of Art*. Grand Rapids: Baker Academic.
Taves, Ann. (1999) *Fits, Trances, and Visions: Experiencing Religion and Explaining Experience from Wesley to James*. Princeton, NJ: Princeton University Press.
Thoreau, Henry David. (2009) *The Journals of Henry David Thoreau, 1837-1861*. New York, NY: Review of Books Classics.

Philip Salim Francis is a professor of philosophy and religion in his home state at the University of Maine-Farmington and Director of Seguinland Institute. His book, *When Art Disrupts Religion: Aesthetic Experience and the Evangelical Mind*, was published by Oxford University Press in 2017. After teaching at Carleton College and Manhattan College, he was a Mellon Fellow in the Humanities at the University of Pennsylvania in 2016. His work has appeared in the *Harvard Theological Review*, *The Atlantic* and the *LA Review of Books*. He teaches courses on religion, aesthetics and back-to-the-land spirituality.

Chapter 11

Seeing the Gods: Divine Embodiment through Visualisation in Tantric Buddhist Practice

DAWN H. COLLINS

This chapter will explore notions of seeing in Buddhism with a focus on the visions and visualisations found in tantric practices and how these engender deity embodiment as lived reality. Sight in tantric Buddhism is, in effect, blind-sighted. This is because to visualise does not require the physical ability to see. In fact, during the death process, so vital for the direction of reincarnation, the practitioner's deity yoga, involving single-pointed concentration on the tutelary deity and absorption of the deity is an internal process not reliant on (often failing) physical sight. In visualisation one's seeing is internal, subtle. The starting point for it may be hearing words about the appearance of the deity and/or the eyes gazing upon an image or statue of the deity figure, but the sight is then internalised and takes place on a much subtler level than physical seeing: the level of the yogic, subtle body. Ultimately, Buddhist thought holds that mind and form are inextricably interconnected, so visualisation forms the basis for a transformation of the subtle aggregates of being such that a new tantric reality emerges; an embodied divinity. Such visualisations, within the context of deity yoga practice, can create visions—both dreaming and waking—of deity worlds. The practitioner's experience of the world is transformed through visualisation such that this subtler reality ceases to become a visualisation and instead is lived as 'real' by those practitioners who have accomplished such profound psychophysical transformation. This type of 'seeing' in Buddhism thus transforms the practitioner's psychophysical aggregates and, in doing so, their lived realities. It is also thought to give them the ability to transform the worlds of those around them, since such practitioners are credited with enhanced abilities to affect the lives of others through their relationship with deity worlds. The present chapter will explore how this plays out in the case of one such tantric practitioner on the Tibetan Plateau, the Pelden Lawa of Rebgong.

Vision according to Buddhist thought is founded on one of six sense bases (P. *āyatana*),[1] or foundations in the senses. The act of seeing is both based in the eye faculty and simultaneously an act of consciousness. It is the same for all other 'sense doors' through which consciousnesses arise: hearing, tasting, touching, smelling and thinking. The early Buddhist textual traditions of the Theravāda Pāli Canon are contained in a tripartite division of 'baskets' (P. *piṭaka*): collections of narrative teachings (P. *sutta*), discourses on the monastic way of life (P. *vinaya*), and systematic theoretical exposition of Buddhist thought, or 'higher teaching' (P. *abhidhamma*). The Pāli literature can be broadly structured around seven core themes, of which the sense faculties are one, and this forms the frame for the epistemological works of the *abhidhamma* (Gethin 2001: 21–22), which further divides these into detailed subcategories.

CONTEMPLATIVE SEEING

In exploring vision in the context of Buddhist practice, I would like to highlight here its role in contemplation. One of the major collections of texts of the Pāli Canon, the *Dīgha Nikāya*, contains a discourse on mindfulness known as the *Mahāsatipaṭṭhānasutta*. Here, in the section concerning the sense bases, we read:

> ...a monk abides contemplating mind-objects as mind-objects in respect of the six internal and external sense bases. How does he do so? Here a monk knows the eye, knows sight objects, and he knows whatever fetter arises dependent on the two. (Walshe 1995: 342)

As can be seen here, the foundation of vision is twofold; the sense faculty is understood to include the 'internal' aspect, meaning the eye itself, and the 'external' aspect, meaning the eye's objects, external forms; vision entails an inextricable relationship between seeing and its object. Through contemplation of this in respect of all the senses, Buddhism posits that

---

1 All non-English terms in brackets will be labelled as follows: P: Pāli; S: Sanskrit; T: Tibetan. Tibetan terms will be transliterated using the Wylie system of transliteration.

their six doors can be closed, leading ultimately to liberation from the fetters binding us to continual rebirth in an unenlightened, cyclical existence (S. *saṃsāra*); in other words, to enlightenment (P. *nibbāna*; S. *nirvāṇa*).

The essential motif of this enlightened vision is that the mediator understands there is no self in the seeing, no doer outside of the conglomerate of aggregates (including the sense faculties) constituting 'a being,' and no object of seeing either. All components of the universe (P. *dhamma*) interdependently arise and dissolve in a state of constant change. No person who sees, nor object seen, has any inherently enduring selfhood or essence. A person who leaves the householder life in search of liberation from the round of rebirth and takes up the life of a homeless wanderer is thus described metaphorically as 'not being bound to the impressions of the six senses' (Collins 1982: 169). Therefore, the meditator who goes to the forest, the root of a tree or an empty place, considers 'eye is not-self, as are material objects, the ear and sounds, the nose and smells, the body and what is tangible, the mind and mental objects' (Collins 1982: 114, drawing on the *Atharva Veda* 109).

This type of contemplative 'seeing' became thematic throughout developments in Buddhist philosophic discourse, particularly after the early first century work of Nāgārjuna, who is credited with originating the influential Mahāyāna school of philosophy known as the school of the 'Middle Way' (Madhyamaka), and whose salient legacy is his deconstructionist 'emptiness' (S. *śūnyatā*); the realisation of how things and events truly exist. In his elucidating work on 'seeing' in a Buddhist philosophic sense, Malcolm David Eckel chooses as his lens the work of the sixth century Madhayamaka philosopher Bhāvaviveka. Following Collins (1982: 3), his rational for this choice rests not only on Bhāvaviveka's philosophic rigour and insight, but on his eloquent use of metaphor 'to bring the complex and abstract concepts of Buddhist Philosophy down to earth' (Eckel 1992: 2). Indeed, the notion of metaphor itself, as word-picture, could be considered allegoric for Buddhist notions of vision, entailing as they do a sense of bodily eye function, the act of seeing and perception of object as mutually arising parts to a non-substantial whole. Contemplative seeing not only enables philosophic insight but Buddhist thought holds that it can lead to the 'direct perception' of an absent Buddha; an ultimate reality. This notion is imbued with a visual aspect in that such perception of how things and events actually exist enable visions and even embodiments of other realms. It is this type of seeing that the esoteric Buddhist systems explore in the visualisations of tantric deity yoga practices.

The continual contemplation of representations of deities such as this Medicine Buddha (**Figure 11.1**) is foundational to the revelatory visions reported throughout Buddhist mythohistories. As Eckel observes, the process of visualisation entailed in esoteric Buddhist systems can produce an experience which is reportedly one wherein absorption can be so deep that the practitioner loses all awareness of surroundings, yet sensory experience is enhanced (Eckel 1992: 134). The type of vision described here is one in which 'seeing' is taking place with an inner eye whose ability to paint in vibrantly emotive imagery is far more advanced than the bodily eye has capacity for.

Here I would like to mention the work of Hugues de Montalembert, a French writer, painter and documentary filmmaker who lost his physical

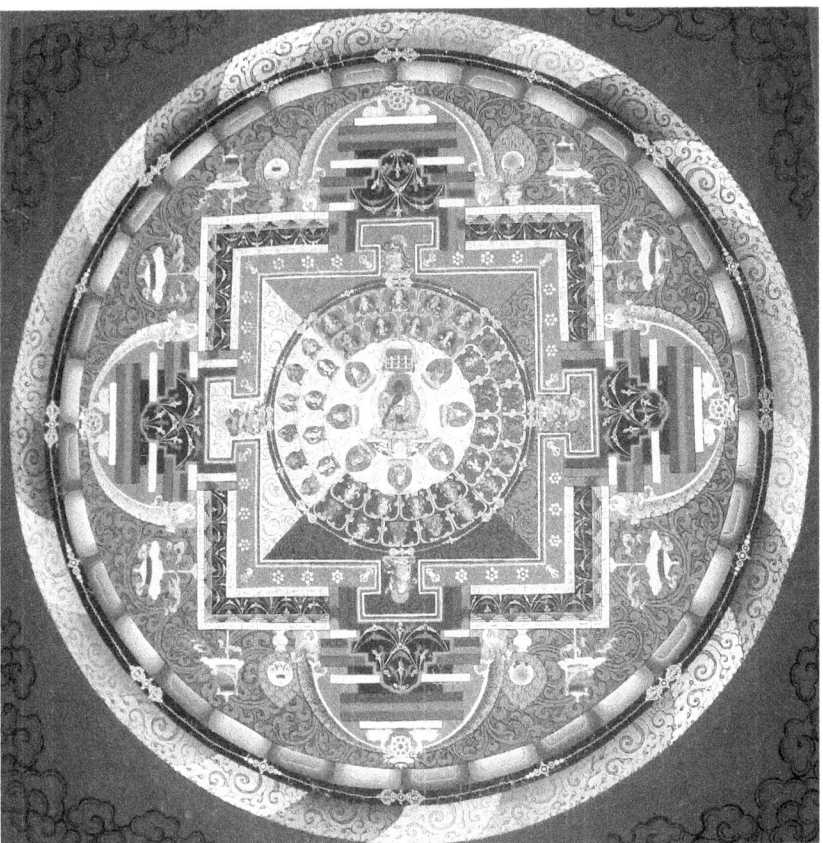

Figure 11.1 A Tibetan silk painting (T. *thang kha*) depicting the divine realm (S. *maṇḍala*) of the Medicine Buddha. Photo by Dawn H. Collins.

sight in a New York apartment burglary in 1978. He has since written an acclaimed autobiographical book, *Eclipse* (1985), which describes the process of becoming blinded and the journey towards publishing his written work. Eight years after his 'blinding,' he said in an interview that he sees so clearly when he writes that, sometimes, when he becomes tired and stops writing, he finds himself looking around, blaming his glasses for his sudden lack of vision.[2] In *Eclipse* and the subsequent film based on his work, *Black Sun* (2005),[3] he explores experiences of vision that are clearly non-sight-dependent in the types of ways pointed towards by Buddhist philosophers. In an interview with his publisher, he says:

> You don't necessarily have a vision. Maybe you have only a perception. And I came to the point that probably to see, to see really, is a creation. And if you speak with painters or architects, it's very strongly there that vision is a creation. (Hugues de Montalembert, interview with Simon and Schuster Books, February 2010)[4]

SEEING DIVINE REALMS

Following Buddhist thought regarding the sense faculties as described in Tibetan cultural contexts, it does not make sense to talk of the body or matter in separation from heart-mind; the world around us, the perceiver and the perceived arise in symbiotic non-dual moments of experience. This thinking has underpinned much of scholarship in this area and is in keeping with tantric notions of the universe. Samuel described this orientation as 'mind-body-world' (Samuel 2001). Craig uses a common anthropological model in referring to it as 'biopsychosocial,' reflecting that 'environment' in this context includes beings (Craig 2012). These beings encompass a range of deity and spirit forces who animate the landscape to form distinct ecologies. A world of deities and other spirit beings have

---

2 From an article in *People* by Joshua Hammer, 18 February 1986 (https://people.com/archive/injured-in-a-1978-mugging-artist-hugues-de-montalembert-finds-hope-and-light-in-his-blindness-vol-25-no-7/, last accessed 13 April 2019).
3 The filmmaker Gary Tarn produced a film based on *Eclipse* (1985) in collaboration with Hugues de Montalembert, called *Black Sun* (2005). See http://www.imdb.com/title/tt0478101/, last accessed 13 April 2019.
4 Hugues de Montalembert, interview with his publisher Simon and Schuster Books, February 2010 (https://www.youtube.com/watch?v=68vSVilenMs, last accessed 13 April 2019).

inhabited Tibetan landscapes since as far back as it is possible historically to trace peoples self-designating with Tibetan identities (cf. Van Schaik 2013 [2011]). They play an important role in terms of the meanings that rituals hold for the peoples of Tibetan regions. One such ritual is that of the Leru (T. *klu rol*), particular to Rebgong where I undertook my doctoral

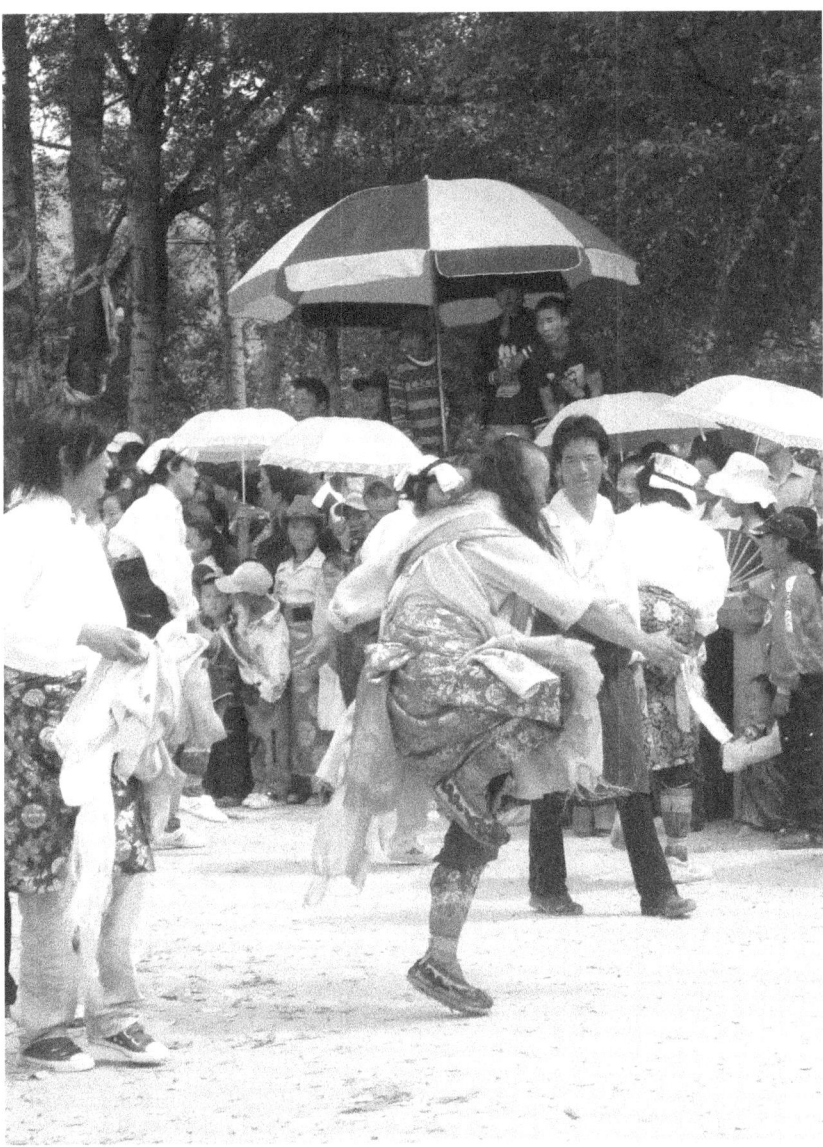

Figure 11.2 Rebgong spirit-medium (*lawa*) at the Leru. Photo by Dawn H. Collins.

fieldwork,[5] and oriented to the mountain gods and other local deities such as the *le* (T. *klu*), serpent deities of the underworlds. The Leru could be described as a ritual based upon a shamanic idiom in which the deity is called down into the person of the spirit-medium, a *lawa* (T. *lha pa*), through possession (**Figure 11.2**). In this type of ritual, the participants 'see' the deity through the person of the *lawa* whose body becomes the instrument of the divine force inhabiting it.

Such shamanic paradigms are often presented in anthropological literature as contrasted with an idiom of specialist rituals, such as the tantric rituals found in Tibetan cultural regions, in which the deity is evoked rather than called down through possession. As with the Leru and its shamanic idiom, the participation in group tantric rituals is thought to enhance well-being. Benefits such as the promotion of health and longevity, healing illness and protection from harm are thought to accrue not only to those directly facilitating the ritual but to its spectators. Such benefits are referred to in Tibetan as descending from the gods, literally 'blessings descend,' *chinbab* (T. *chin babs*).

The deity yoga practised by Tibetan tantric adepts, *nukwa* (T. *sngags pa*),[6] in direct contrast to the type of shamanic idiom of a *lawa*, is a highly structured and controlled affair (**Figure 11.3**). An assortment of parallel innovations in Indian Śaivite and Mahāyāna Buddhist traditions from the seventh century onward gradually became labelled '*tantra*' and formed the basis for tantric Buddhism (S. *vajrayāna*) as received and now practised among Tibetan communities. This emergent Vajrayāna Buddhism drew on the deity visualisation practices of the Mahāyāna Buddhism already established by the sixth century (Samuel 2008: 291). As discussed, these were underpinned by a contemplative 'seeing' based in the philosophical thought attributed to Indian philosophers such as Nāgārjuna. The practices of Indian *siddha* adepts, from whom the Vajrayāna tantric practice found in Tibetan regions can be said to originate (cf. Samuel 2005: 57), underlie a meditative practice involving the transformation of individuals and their environs into deities and deity abodes (S. *maṇḍala*) respectively. Tantric practice usually involves the recitation of texts. Texts in contemporary Tibetan cultural regions are vital. They are embodied in the way in which they are chanted out loud; voiced into being by the practitioners

5 The Rebgong Valley is located in China's Qinghai Province and sits on the northeastern Tibetan Plateau to the south side of the Yellow River.
6 The phonetic rendition of this term '*nukwa*' follows a pronunciation used in the region of the ethnographic section to follow.

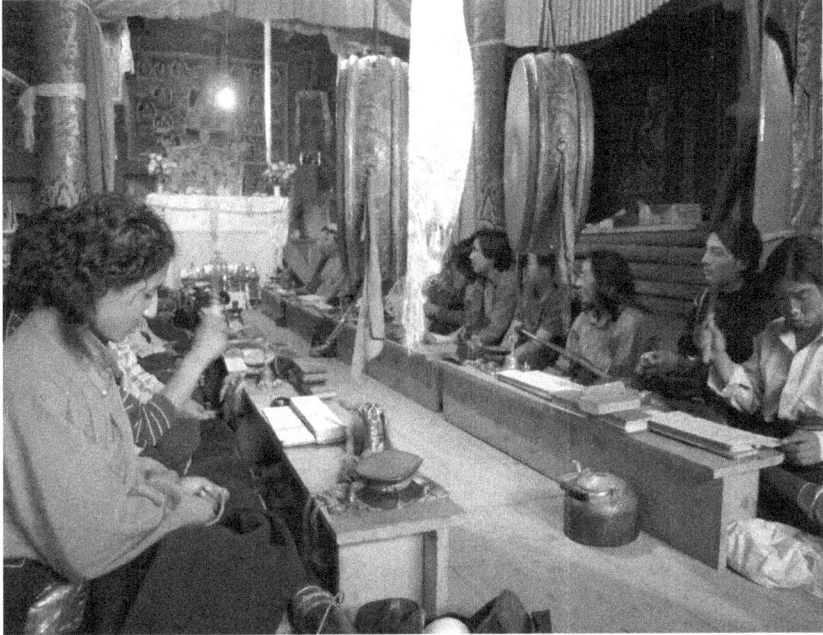

Figure 11.3 Tantric practitioners in Rebgong. Photo by Dawn H. Collins.

who seek to evoke deity and spirit worlds in doing so. Texts thus form part of living traditions designed to (re)create the presence of deity worlds and the embodied landscapes they (re)create as sacred.

The different tantric *sādhana*, or 'practice manuals,' found across Tibetan Buddhist traditions require having received initiation from a qualified teacher, a *lama*. Indeed, the initiation ritual itself may be considered a *sādhana* in that the *lama* concerned performs a ritual self-initiation as deity, following the format of *sādhana*, as preparation for bestowing this on others.[7] Hence, an outline of the *sādhana* format will provide insight into the elements designating it as *tantric*.

The main visualisation processes involving the evocation of the deity are preceded by preliminaries purifying or establishing the place for the ritual, and followed by the dissolution of visualisations and other concluding rites. The 'one who practices the *sādhana*' (S. *sādhaka*) may begin by generating self as a wrathful deity who dispels all obstacles to the successful completion of the ritual, thereby purifying the place. S/he then

---

7 The *lama* performs multiple roles within this ritual as guide, even taking into account what dreams occur as part of his ritual role (Lamb 1994: 23).

protects that ritual arena with a visualised *vajra*[8] tent. Preliminaries may include the generation of motivational intent accompanied by activities to prepare the *sādhaka*, such as recitation of the refuge formula and prostrations. They may also entail the setting of the philosophical scene in terms of recollection of the 'four abidings' and 'emptiness' (S. *śūnyatā*), which are the basis for the realisation of means and wisdom respectively. Preliminary offerings may be made to the teachers of the lineage, emphasising the importance of devotion to the *lama* who gave initiation into the *tantra*, and to the host of deities to be invoked.

The deities are visualised as emerging from within their envisaged palace, or *maṇḍala*. They are created firstly as pledge-beings (S. *samayasattva*), which are then consecrated by the evocation of their respective knowledge-beings (S. *jñānasattva*) from out of 'emptiness,' utilising light from their seed syllables (S. *bīja*), which are invited to become inseparable from them. At this point, the deity, whether seen as before the *sādhaka*, or seen *as* the *sādhaka*, is considered to be actually present. Praises, offerings and requests are then made to the deity, accompanied by ritual hand gestures (S. *mudrā*). This second phase can be viewed, in some *sādhana*, as the 'completion stage,' the stages prior to this being termed the 'generation stage' of the practice. The recitation of *mantra* may be accompanied by various practices of breath control designed to harness the energy winds flowing along the channels and *cakra* of the subtle body. It is, therefore, on the basis of the corporal body that the subtle levels of being are transformed, and on the basis of this that the practitioner will come to embody the deity s/he contemplates. In the completion stage *sādhana*, these breath control yoga practices are subdivided into those 'with sign' and those without, the 'sign' being the *maṇḍala* of the deity and its inhabitants.

The concluding rites include dispersing the wisdom-beings and the absorption of the pledge-being by the *sādhaka*, before specific requests and aspirations are laid before the deities on the premise that, should the ritual have been successfully accomplished, they are obliged to grant these. At the conclusion of the completion stage *sādhana*, the *sādhaka* arises as the deity from a 'signless' yoga (Skorupski 2002). At the highest levels of tantric practice, it is taught that the prerequisite for completion stage yoga is the ability at generation stage to be able to hold a complete and detailed visualisation of the deity's form, *maṇḍala* and retinue, in the size

---

8 The *vajra*, as the ritual implement that has come to symbolise Tantric Buddhism, is the embodiment of its power and represents 'means' [the bell, with which it is usually held in practice, represents its counterpart: 'wisdom' (S. *prajñā*)].

of the head of a pin, for four hours straight in complete absorption. As can be seen, in tantric deity yoga practice, it is through visualisations of deities and their abodes that the practitioner either becomes, unifies with or realises true nature as deity. The ability to generate such visualisations through intensive practice in contemplative seeing is thus the foundation for enlightenment according to a Buddhist tantric understanding. These same meditative techniques are applied during the death process to enable liberation from unenlightened existence and the cycle of rebirth, since the death process is an opportunity, as the vision of this life fades, to transform one's vision of existence. The practitioner's deity yoga, involving single-pointed concentration on tutelary deity and absorption of deity is an internal process not reliant on an (often failing) physical sight (cf. Coleman 2006). Ultimately, in Buddhist thought, we are enlightened, if we could only see it. Therefore, tantric practices aim, through the transformation of the senses and an internalisation of seeing via contemplation and visualisation, to create the practitioner's world as that of deity. As will be seen in the ethnography to follow below, those who have accomplished this acquire the ability to transform those around them and their environs. The ethnography describes how a tantric adept uses such visionary practices to evoke the presence of the deity Palden Lhamo, yet in this rite not as tantric tutelary deity but as the deity ruling his subtle body's energetic channels, in an act of embodiment characterised as mediumship, i.e. as a *lawa*.

EMBODIED VISIONS

In the ethnography below, this Rebgong adept, famous in the traditional Amdo region[9] of the Tibetan Plateau for his ability to heal, would become possessed not by a mountain deity but by a deity of the entourage of the powerful Buddhist protector deity Palden Lhamo (T. dPal ldan lha mo). It is hardly surprising that an adept *nukwa*, a tantric practitioner who embodies such deities during yogic practice and then in addition is able to become possessed by Palden Lhamo or her retinue during a ritual for healing the sick, would be much in demand amongst Tibetan communities, as was the case with the *nukwa lawa* here. This *nukwa* was reputedly a very powerful

---

9 The term Amdo refers to a historical Tibetan regional division of the Plateau into the tripartite provinces (T. *chol kha gsum*) of Ütsang, Kham and Amdo (T. dBus gtsang, Khams and A mdo).

healer, known for his healing powers not only as a *nukwa* but as a *lawa*, and because of this is known locally as the Pelden Lawa.¹⁰ He was attributed the ability to 'see' in a clairvoyant, divinatory sense, and also with the deep knowledge of contemplative seeing that comes with being a tantric adept.

Palden Lhamo is important in various ways throughout Tibetan regions in different contexts. She is a major focus of national identity as the wrathful protector deity of the Tibetans and the Dalai Lama, the Gelukpa (T. dGe lugs pa)¹¹ rulers of Tibetan regions in a reincarnation lineage since the mid-seventeenth century. Veneration of her is not limited to Buddhists, since she is a straight adaptation of the pre-Buddhist Bön deity Sipéjelmo (T. Srid pa'i gyal mo), one of the major Bön deities. To the Bön, Sipéjelmo is known as the 'Queen of the World,' having birthed twenty-seven daughters from eggs, nine of them central in her entourage. She is consort to a variety of tantric deities and a protector deity with nine hundred heads, one thousand arms and a chameleon-like complexion said to change six times in every twenty-four hours. It is said that 'half the sky is her canopy and half the earth is her mate'¹² (Karmay, 2013: 20–21).

In one of their most commonly known aspects, both Sipéjelmo and Palden Lhamo ride a mule, as shown in the image here (**Figure 11.4**). Palden Lhamo is accorded a high status within Buddhism as supreme protector, and her power is considered much greater than that of the local deities and spirits. She is venerated by a large number of people in Tibetan cultural regions as attested to by the proliferation of her images and communal observances.¹³ Palden Lhamo, apart from being Buddhism's most important protector, is also known for her clairvoyant powers and ability in divination. It was traditionally through recourse to her divinatory powers that successive reincarnations of the Dalai Lama were determined. Lhamolhatso is her sacred lake and it was in its waters that these visionary divinations of future Dalai Lama were sought by those seeking to maintain

10 This is a pseudonym. The *nukwa* was particularly concerned to preserve his anonymity and I promised to do so as far as possible, hence I have not included details of his native village, etc. anywhere in my research.
11 The Gelukpa school of Tibetan Buddhism, whose founder Tsongkhapa (T. Tsong kha pa) was born near modern-day Xining, first began to establish itself in Rebgong early in the seventeenth century (Dhondup 2011: 42).
12 '*gnam phyed bla yi khebs / sa phyed 'od gi gdam*' (translation Karmay 2013).
13 I was fortunate to experience myself in both 2006 and 2007 an annual Lhasa festival day held in her honour. in which her images are particularly venerated and women can be made offerings to as sacred reflections of the protector goddess.

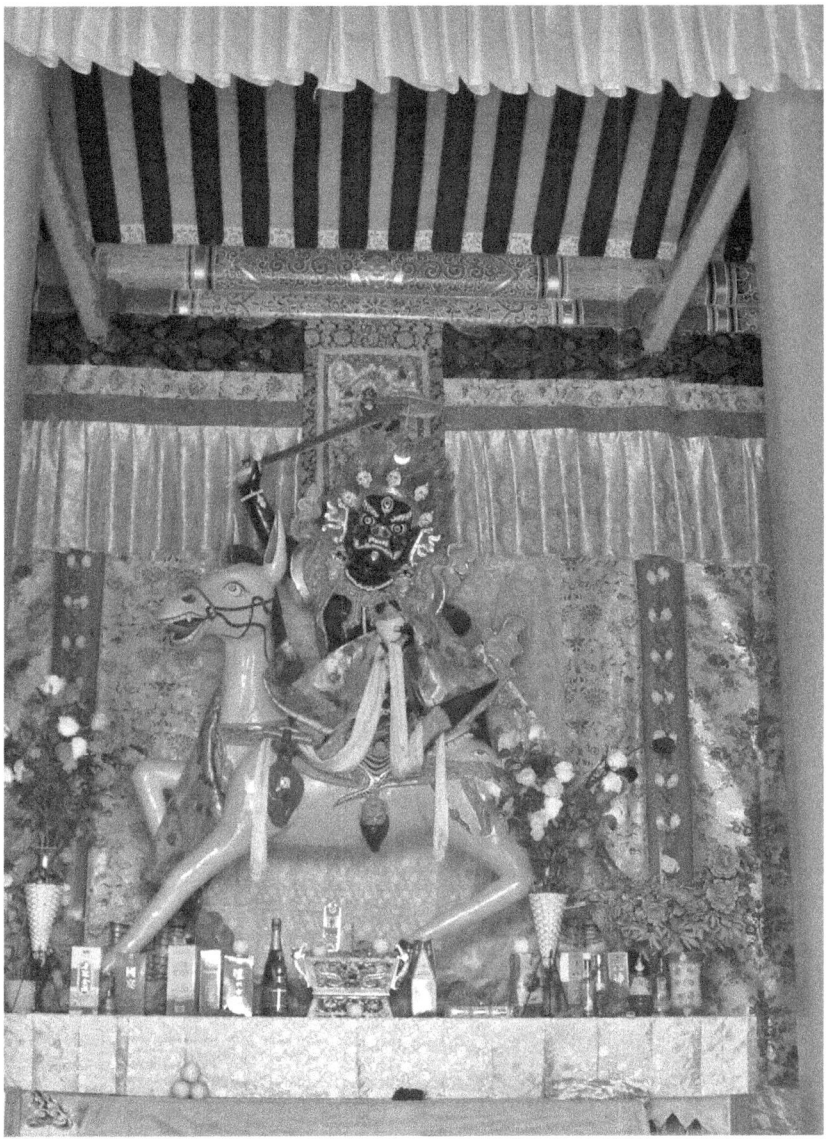

Figure 11.4 Palden Lhamo statue in a Rebgong temple for the local deities. Photo by Dawn H. Collins.

the line of reincarnatory succession (Goldstein 1989: 310ff). The lake is a major pilgrimage site and many travel there hoping to receive a blessing or vision from its waters (**Figure 11.5**). Those pilgrims who make the journey will often spend hours sitting beside the lake or on the mountains

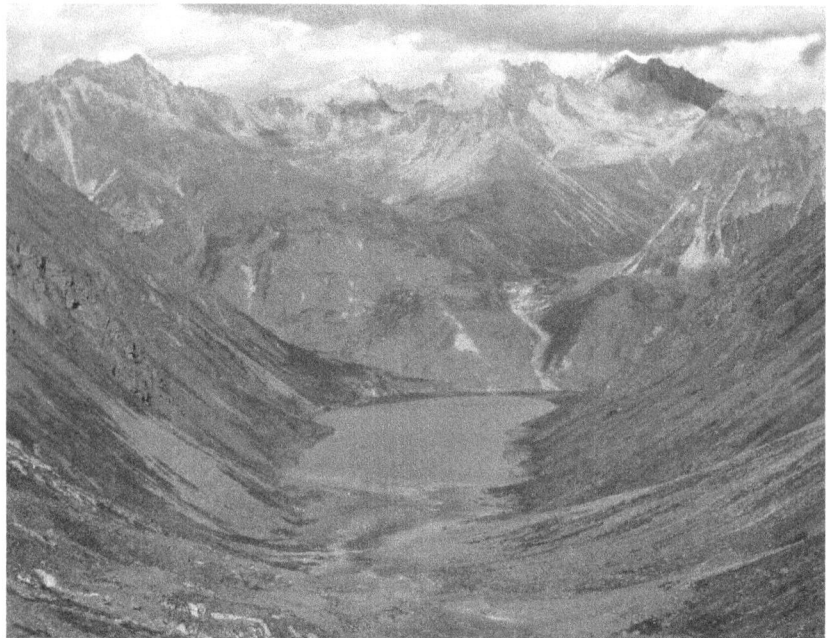

Figure 11.5 Lhamolhatso Lake. Photo by Dawn H. Collins.

above it, praying for such a vision. This implies the belief that a non-sight-dependent seeing can arise due to blessing from a divine power at a location in the natural world especially linked to that power. Sitting there for hours listening to the sound of *mantra* chanting by the pilgrims awaiting such blessed vision, it is clear that this is perceived as perfectly possible.[14]

Palden Lhamo's power in divination extends beyond mundane affairs in that she is said to be able to predict karmic outcomes for an individual; something ordinarily only considered possible for an enlightened being in the context of Buddhism (Beer 2003: 156–159). Her mythohistory has her taking the life of her son in order to protect Buddhism, after clairvoyantly perceiving the threat he would pose to it should she not do so. This ability in clairvoyance makes her practice particularly helpful in the divinatory treatment of disease. As can be seen from the above, the ability to 'see' here includes non-sight-dependent visions in water and clairvoyant 'seeing' the future. These types of non-ordinary seeing are interwoven with the capacity to divine and to heal, intrinsic to both of which is the ability to 'see' karmic outcomes.

14 This was my sense from visiting Lhamolhatso in September 2006.

It is worth noting here the significance of *karma* in ways of seeing. According to a Buddhist view, insofar as we are unenlightened, we are all reincarnated in an endless cycle of becoming in which the aspects of being which pass from life to life are attached to numerous bodies in the course of their rebirths. Past thought-actions and present mental states create karmic winds, propelling continuums of being into rebirth as spider, fly, bird, elephant, dolphin, bee, human, *nāga*, hell-being, demon, tree-spirit, and so on. The physiological aspects of sight are affected by bodily capacities, such as having eight eyes, the capacity to see colour or polarised light. To know what others see is an experiential impossibility, as Adrian Horridge eloquently expressed in relation to the honeybee:

> However deep our understanding, we will never know every detail of the bee's visual system, or that of any other simple brain, because...we...omit the essential settings of the gain, noise, time constants, feedback loops, ionic changes and hormonal effects, as well as the processes of growth and decay that all contribute to neural activity. (Horridge 2009: xv)

In short, only those with the karmic propensities resultant in rebirth as a bee can know what it is to see as a bee. In the same way, the aspects of sight which involve consciousness are karmically propelled to discriminate on the basis of physiological vision. For example, in the case of the subjective ability to 'see' beauty. As the ancient Greek poet Sappho said,

> Some say thronging cavalry, some say foot soldiers, others call a fleet the most beautiful of sights the dark earth offers, but I say it's whatever you love best. (Powell [trans.] 2007: 6–7)

The way in which a being sees is dependent on bodily formations, mental formations and, ultimately, the karmic winds which guide these towards perceptions of self and the world. Buddhist thought holds that through practices such as those of tantric deity yoga, these aspects of sight can be transformed, as per the karmic propensities to reproduce them. This results in an increasingly subtle relation to self and the divine, in which one's perception of self and world become aligned to the divine; to a clear vision of the world in ultimate terms. Enlightenment is not only to see the gods but to see as them; the ability to see and know oneself, the natural world and its beings from the perspective of profound insight into the actual nature of all.

To return to the healer of the ethnographic account to follow, the Pelden Lawa had a special reputation for curing illness precisely because of his reputation as such an adept; combining the abilities of a high-level tantric practitioner and *lawa*; someone who can see the gods and, in some profound sense, see and heal as them. Many Rebgong residents told me they were acquainted with somebody who had been assisted by him. I was told that his 'cures' involved performing physical feats under possession that would not be possible under normal conditions: in this case, piercing his tongue with a metal spike or stirring boiling oil with his bare hands. I was not privy to any such dramatic events with this *lawa*, who was quite reticent initially about talking to me at all. However, I include here a brief ethnography describing one ritual healing performed by the Pelden Lawa, with assistance from several *nukwa*, which he permitted me to attend during the course of my fieldwork. This ritual was hosted in a sponsor's house, borrowed for the occasion, since a good deal of space was needed to accommodate all the parties involved. My account begins in that household's large walled courtyard in Torjia (T. Tho gyal) county.[15]

The sick man entered the dusty courtyard supported by a man on either side. He attempted to place one foot in front of the other but his legs kept buckling underneath him. His clothes were dirty and dishevelled. He and his brothers had travelled far to see the Pelden Lawa, who would perform a ritual hoped to be of powerful benefit for the sick man's health. It had been more than a year that Tenzin could hardly walk. He was not yet even forty years old, yet he was semi-paralysed and crippled with pain. His brothers had taken him to their nearest State biomedical hospital, where the doctors had been unable to help. His relatives had even taken him to Lhasa, to the traditional Tibetan medicine hospital (T. *sMan rtsis khang*), but to no avail.

After they had deposited Tenzin inside the house on a bed in the room where the ritual would take place, the brothers joined me on wooden benches in the courtyard where butter tea was being served for the various people peripheral to the ritual. The brothers started to talk about their hopes for the ritual healing.[16] Three donkeys arrived with provisions and the *nukwa*'s trusted assistants rushed in and out unloading the donkeys

15 All the information contained in this account was collected through unstructured interviews in my limited Amdo dialect with those involved in the rites. Separate interviews with the Pelden Lawa were conducted both before and after the ritual. One of these was conducted via an interpreter translating to Lhasa dialect. I am indebted to Nicholas Silhé for joining me at this interview and kindly sharing his transcripts.
16 All information about the case of this man, given the pseudonym Tenzin, and the ritual performed for his health, is taken from notes made during fieldwork conducted in Rebgong during 2009, unless otherwise stated.

Visualisation in Tantric Buddhist Practice 215

and galvanising others into action preparing the space. After the donkeys had been unloaded and the courtyard was peaceful again, I forced down another mouthful of butter tea and waited for the brothers to resume. They began recounting an oral history demonstrating the reputed power of the Pelden Lawa which had drawn them to this place. In the early 1980s, 'Wenchen Rinpoché,' the tenth in the line of incarnations of the Panchen Lama, and second only in lamaic status to the Dalai Lama, had visited the area. Many of the local *lawa* had gone into possession, channelling the local mountain deities to greet this high Buddhist *lama*. However, since these deities were local deities, they could not approach the Panchen Lama because of his Buddhist refuge and the power of his practice. In contrast, when the Pelden Lawa came towards the Panchen Lama in full possession, he presented an offering scarf in full view of everyone. This story was concrete proof for Tenzin's brothers of the Pelden Lawa's powers. As they began reminiscing in their dialect, I escaped to the preparation room before another butter tea was offered to me.

The room in which the preparations for the Jelwa ritual (T. bsGral ba) were almost complete was wall-papered with toy rabbits holding balloons **(Figure 11.6)**. They smiled down on all the flags depicting the lords of

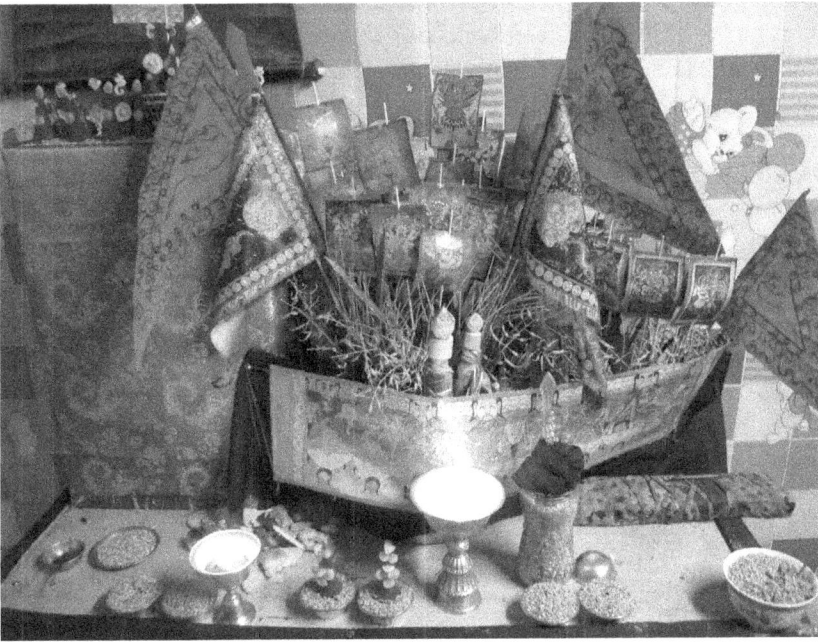

Figure 11.6 Shurwu Tongdok ritual offerings. Photo by Dawn H. Collins.

sickness in eerie dissonance. The Jelwa can be a family or village ritual, but in the case of Tenzin, since his illness was so severe, it needed to be the large Jelwa by a practitioner as powerful as the Pelden Lawa to stand any chance of having an effect. It was a purification ritual to clear the sick man's channels (T. *rtsa*) of the malevolent spirits possessing him. This type of ritual was the forté of the Pelden Lawa, who travelled far and wide on demand to help those afflicted with various types of illnesses believed to have been caused by spirit harm. He made a living from this practice, both for himself and the entourage of younger *nukwa* who assisted him. He gave a portion of the money donated to him by the families of those he healed to the community of *nukwa* to which he belonged, and was also using a portion to assist in rebuilding a local *nukwa* temple.

As later explained in interview with the Pelden Lawa, via a translator, the particular Jelwa ritual to be performed for Tenzin's benefit was called Shurwu Tongdok (T. Phur pu gtong 'dogs). In it the Pelden Lawa would became possessed, not by a mountain deity but by a deity of the entourage of the powerful Buddhist protector deity Palden Lhamo. This deity, the ruler of the Pelden Lawa's channels or *tsadak* (T. *rtsa bdag*), is known as Chötsen Donchen (T. Chu srin gdong can), the Crocodile Faced One. She and the rather better-known Sengé Donchen (T. Seng ge gdong can) regularly accompany Palden Lhamo. Both these female attendants of Palden Lhamo are animal-headed. Chötsen Donchen, who has the head of a *makara*, is the *ḍākinī* on Palden Lhamo's right. She wears a human skin, holds a noose or snare in her right hand and the reins of Palden Lhamo's mule in her left, as can be seen in the illustration here. The more well-known *ḍākinī*, Sengé Donchen, has a lion's head, and is seen at Palden Lhamo's left. She is red in colour and holds a noose and a skull cup (**Figure 11.7**).[17]

In the Shurwu Tongdok ritual, and typically for healing rituals conducted by the Pelden Lawa, he creates drawn effigies of all the harmful agents, the spirit beings, lords of sickness (T. *nad bdag*) attacking the patient. Once the Pelden Lawa has been entered by Chötsen Donchen and so filled with the power of this deity, with the other deities of Palden Lhamo's entourage lending their support, each drawn effigy is burnt and the ash thrown into boiling oil which the Pelden Lawa reportedly stirs with his bare hands. In accordance with a characteristic description of *dulwa*, the Pelden Lawa's own description of this ritual process made the distinction that it was the harm that was ritualistically being destroyed, not the

---

17   http://www.casotac.com/CASonline%20Articles/IMG-20120619-0028221.jpg (last accessed 3 May 2019).

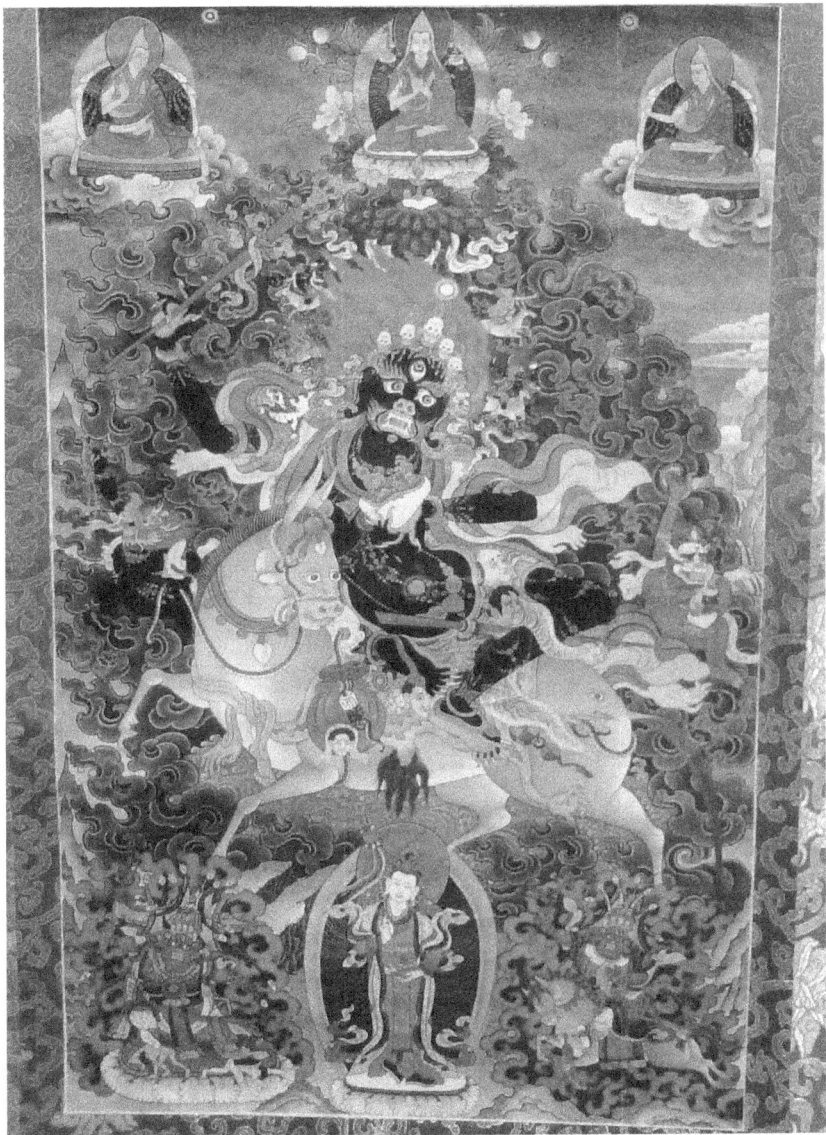

Figure 11.7 A *thang kha* depicting Palden Lhamo with retinue, Chötsen Donchen to her right and Sengé Donchen to her left. Charitable Assistance Society, Phuntsok Cho Ling Buddhist Centre, public domain.

harmful deities themselves. He said he would visualise the harm dissolving and that the fact that it did was due to the blessing, the *chinlab*, of the lama-yidam, the deity of his root tantric practice. At the end of the Shurwu Tongdok, one of the *nukwa* who had been assisting the Pelden Lawa came to tell Tenzin's brothers that the dream signs were good and so the ritual had been effective.

The case of the Pelden Lawa is the only case I have come across in Rebgong in which one individual performs the function of both a tantric practitioner, a *nukwa*, and a *lawa*, a spirit-medium. One explanation or frame for why this is possible in his particular case could lie in the fact that the deity he embodies as spirit-medium is from the entourage of a high Buddhist protector deity, and so not in precisely the same order of beings as the mountain deities who are *tsadak* (channels) of most, if not all, other spirit-mediums in Rebgong. The Buddhist protector deities are considered as primarily concerned with other-worldly goals in that, if not enlightened, they are at least upholding enlightenment as the goal and protecting practitioners towards that end, rather than being primarily concerned with things of this life, such as protecting crops and so forth. In the case of the Pelden Lawa, the deity is perceived to work through him, one individual, as both Buddhist tantric practitioner and spirit-medium. It could be said that the deities work through the tantric practitioners, whose practice has brought them to a state in which they embody the deities they invoke. This transmitted healing derives from an empowerment from the deity, a blessing descending through the practitioner's deity yoga, key to which is a contemplative seeing; a visualisation process resultant in embodiment.

This aspect of seeing in Buddhist thought and practice is the inner seeing of our dreams and visions. It is broadly founded on theories of non-self, wherein the faculty of the eye is understood as encompassing seeing and its object as mutually arising and intrinsically empty of any permanent, substantial entity. As such, the sense sphere of the eye is, as with other sense spheres, a door to awareness. Seeing transforms with awareness. Key to this, from early Buddhism through to present-day lived religious practice, is the meditative act of contemplating the sense doors. This contemplative seeing, developed through practice, is non-sight-dependent, illuminating the object of sight with mind. Just as for a blind person there is still a form of seeing, the development of this inner vision prepares the ground for a clearer awareness; for seeing the true nature of things and events. A process of developing visualisation practice on the basis of this contemplative ability and its insights is core to the esoteric deity yoga practices of tantric Buddhism. Sight in tantric Buddhism, in effect, is blind-sighted because to visualise does not require the physical ability to see. In visualisation one's seeing is internal, subtle, creating one's seeing anew from within. The type of vision developed through these practices is what we experience in dreams when our bodily eyes are closed, and during the death process, and it is reported by religious adepts across multiple religions when they speak of seeing waking visions. Bringing this theoretical frame into a lived reality in a Tibetan Buddhist community, as exemplified in the above ethnography, an adept with high levels of ability to 'see' deity worlds becomes them. Through this embodiment deity worlds become a lived reality and the practitioner is understood as able to transform the 'seeing' of those around; to cause others to see differently; to heal and to be healed.

REFERENCES

Beer, R. (2003) *The Handbook of Tibetan Symbols*. Boston: Shambhala Publications.

Coleman, G. (ed.) with Jinpa, T. and Dorje, G. (trans.) (2006) *The Tibetan Book of the Dead*. New York: Penguin.

Collins, S. (1982) *Selfless Persons: Imagery and thought in Theravāda Buddhism*. Cambridge: University Press. https://doi.org/10.1017/CBO9780511621499

Craig. S. (2012) *Healing Elements: Efficacy and the Social Ecologies of Tibetan Medicine*. Berkeley and London: University of California Press.
https://doi.org/10.1525/california/9780520273238.001.0001

De Montalembert, Hugues. (1985) *Eclipse*, translated by David Noakes. New York: Viking Books.

Dhondup, T. Yangdon. (2011) 'Reb kong: Religion, History and Identity of a Sino-Tibetan borderland town,' *Revue d'Etudes Tibétaines*, 22, November, 33-59.

Eckel, M. D. (1992) *To See the Buddha: A Philosopher's Quest for the Meaning of Emptiness*. New Jersey: Princeton University Press.

Gethin, R. (2001) *The Buddhist Path to Awakening*. Oxford: OneWorld.

Goldstein, M. (1989) *A History of Modern Tibet, 1913-1951: The Demise of the Lamaist State*. Berkeley: University of California Press.

Horridge, A. (2009) *What does the honeybee see and how do we know? A Critique of Scientific Reason*. Canberra: Australian National University E-press.
https://doi.org/10.22459/WHS.10.2009

Karmay, S. G. (2013) 'Queen of the World and Her Twenty-seven Daughters,' *Journal of the International Association for Bon Research*, 1, 21-35.

Lamb, C. (1994) in Holm, J. and Bowker, J. (eds.), *Rites of Passage*. London: Pinter Publishers Ltd.

Powell, J. (trans.) (2007) *The Poetry of Sappho*. Oxford: Oxford University Press.

Samuel, G. (2001) 'Tibetan Medicine in Contemporary India: Theory and Practice,' in Connor, L., and Samuel, G. (eds.), *Healing Powers and Modernity*. London: Bergen and Garvey, pp. 247-269.

Samuel, G. (2005) *Tantric Revisionings: New Understandings of Tibetan Buddhism and Indian Religion*. Farnham, UK: Ashgate.
Samuel, G. (2008) *The Origins of Yoga and Tantra: Indic Religions to the Thirteenth Century*. Cambridge and New York: Cambridge University Press.
https://doi.org/10.1017/CBO9780511818820
Skorupski, T. (2002) *Kriyàsaügraha: Compendium of Buddhist Rituals*. Tring: The Institute of Buddhist Studies.
Van Schaik, S. (2013 [2011]) *Tibet: A History*. London and New York: Yale University Press.
Walshe, M. (1995) *The Long Discourses of the Buddha: A Translation of the Dīgha Nikāya*. Boston: Wisdom Publications.

Dr Dawn H. Collins (Research Fellow of the Foro di Studi Avanzati Gaetano Massa [FSA] Roma) lectures with a focus on Buddhism, Hinduism, Sacred Geography, Dance, and Death Studies. Her doctoral thesis, entitled 'Presence in Tibetan Landscapes: spirited agency and ritual healing in Rebgong,' was underpinned by ethnographic fieldwork on the Tibetan Plateau. Her interest in 'lived religions' is inspired not only by her anthropological experience but by her training and work as a contemporary dancer and practitioner of oriental massage therapies. She has supervised postgraduate students at the London Contemporary Dance School, published on ritual dance, and has worked on research projects ranging from a British Academy funded exploration of contemporary ritual expression in Bhutan to background research for a documentary film about life in the Welsh valleys. She is a member of the British Association for the Study of Religions (BASR), the Complementary Therapists Association (CThA), the International Association for the Study of Traditional Asian Medicine (IASTAM), and belongs to an international Research Group on the Body, Health and Religion (BAHAR).

Index

abstraction (art) 19, 149, 151–152, 154–155
Adams, Doug 19
Alhambra 4
Amazon 8
anasyrma 99–100
animals 1, 23, 72, 75
animism 161, 162, 166, 169–170, 173, 176, 178, 180
apotropaic 87–88, 96–97, 99. 102
Arjuna 3, 4
ashe (also *axe*, *ache*) 122, 123
Augustine, Saint 3
Austen, Jane 31–33

beauty 189–192, 196–197
beelding 150–152, 155, 157
Bertram, Anthony 164, 166–167, 176
Bhagavad Gita 3
Bible 2, 126
    Deuteronomy, book of 2
    Genesis, book of 2
    John, Gospel of 2, 3
    Luke, Gospel of 3
Bob Jones University 182–197
Brazil/Brazilian 122, 127, 128, 132, 134
Buddhism/Buddhist 124, 200–220

Candomblé 128, 132, 133, 135
Cardinal, Roger 162, 163, 166–167, 172, 175, 176, 178
Caribbean 122, 124, 127, 128, 129, 130, 132
Catholicism 8, 185–186

Causey, Andrew 163, 164, 165, 170, 173, 175, 176, 177, 178, 179
Charlie Hebdo 39
child/children 19–22, 146, 182–197
Christianity/Christians 3, 132, 182–197
church 3, 124, 125, 126, 131, 182–197
clairvoyance 115, 117, 210, 212
Classen, Constance 7, 71
creation 2

darśan 6
Darwin, Charles 7
De Stijl 147, 149, 151
desire 193–197
Dewey, John 195–196
divination 210, 212
dreams 9, 21, 74, 75, 163, 164–165, 171, 173, 218, 219
Durkheim, Émile 6

Eck, Diana 6
Eliade, Mircea 3
Elias, Jamal 11
Eliot, George 5–6
enchantment 162, 164, 166, 172, 178
evangelical/evangelicalism 5, 182–197
exorcism 116

fieldwork/ethnography 8, 69–74, 122, 123, 209, 213–214, 219
film 9, 10, 46–66, 69–86, 193–194
Foucault, Michel 28
Freud, Sigmund 7, 100–102, 194–195, 197

Gadamer, Hans-Georg 22
Gaddafi, Muammar 38
Gassner, (Fr.) Johann Joseph 116
Gell, Alfred 11
Gillen, Francis James 10
gorgoneion 96–99, 101–102
Gosse, Edmund 184–185
Goulet, Jean-Guy 9
Greek myth/religion 4, 87–102

Haiti 112, 124, 129
Harvey, Graham xi–xiii, 6, 69, 71, 74,161, 162, 163, 172
healing/healer 78–80, 213–214, 216, 219
Heidegger, Martin 22
Hinduism 3, 6
Horridge, Adrian 213
Howes, David 7

Indigenous peoples
  Africa 9
  Australia 6, 10
  death protocols 47–54, 57–58, 61, 63
  New Zealand (Maori) 77–79
  North America 3, 7, 23: Anishinaabe 55–58, 62, 72, 81–83; Dene (Alaska) 73–75; Diné (Navajo) 47–54; Inuit 75–77; Lakota 74, 82; Mi'kmaq 77
  two-spirit/LGBTQ 47, 51–52, 54–55, 57–63
  visual sovereignty 46–47, 54–55, 63, 81–83
  youth suicide 46–47, 49, 54–59, 61, 63
Islam/Muslims 4, 7, 26–45

Jay, Martin 5
Jesus 2, 3, 196, 200, 205–206
Judaism/Jews 3
Jung, Carl 173, 176

Kandinsky, Wassily 5
karma/karmic 212–213
Klug, Brian 38, 42
Krishna 3

landscapes 73–79, 83,160–181, 205, 207, 220
Leru 205–206
LGBTQ 47, 51–52, 54–55, 57–63
Lofton, Kathryn 11
London 23, 153, 203–204

maṇḍala 72, 203, 206, 208
mantra 72, 208, 212
May, Theresa 37–38
Medicine Buddha 203
meditation 24
Merleau-Ponty, Maurice 7
Meyer, Birgit 11
Mitchell, W. J. T. 11
Modood, Tariq 30, 39
Mondrian, Piet 5, 143–159
Montalembert, Hugues de 203–204, 219
Morgan, David 11, 189, 195
Morphy, Howard 10
Moses 2
mountain god/deity 73, 206, 209, 215, 216, 218
Mulvey, Laura 102
museums 10, 25, 143, 203–204
music 5, 129, 199, 200–202, 204, 208
mystery 164, 167, 170, 176, 178, 180
mysticism 165-6, 169, 173, 176

Nāgārjuna 202, 206
Nash, Paul 5, 160–181
Nehamas, Alexander 196
Neo-Plasticism 149, 150–151, 154
New York City 8, 124, 125, 128, 131, 132, 139, 150, 153
Newman, Barnet 19
Niger 8

ontology 161, 163, 164, 170, 179
Oregon Extension 183–197
Orsi, Robert 8
Ovid 4, 88, 94–95

paganism 161, 162, 166, 171–172, 178
Palden Lhamo 209–210, 216–217

Pāli Canon 201
Pamuk, Orhan 4, 5
possession 9, 12, 14, 86, 122, 123, 128, 130, 132, 138, 140, 206, 214–215
Promey, Sally 11
Pygmalion 93–95

Read, Herbert 170, 171, 172, 176, 179
ritual 9, 122, 123, 127, 128, 132, 133, 138, 206–209, 214–216, 218, 220
Rothko, Mark 19, 189–190
Rushdie, Salman 27

Sacks, Oliver 1
Scarry, Elaine 197
sexual assault 47, 54–55, 57–61, 63
Shaeffer, Francis 185–186
Shaeffer, Franky 185–186
Singer, André 10
sixth sense 115
Spencer, Walter Baldwin 10
spirit manifestation 70–78, 83, 123, 124, 128, 129, 131, 133, 135, 136, 137, 138
spirit-medium 205–6, 218
spiritism/spiritist 124, 132, 133, 134, 137
Stoller, Paul 8, 9, 71
Suger (Abbot) 4

symposium (in Greek culture) 96, 98
synagogue 3
Synott, Anthony 7

Taliban 27, 31–33, 39, 41
tantra/tantric 200–202, 204, 206–210, 213–214, 218, 220
Thomas 2
theosophy/theosophical 144, 146, 151
Tibet/Tibetan 23, 201, 205–207, 209–210, 214, 219–220
touch 6, 19, 70, 93–95, 102, 122, 132
Turner, Edith 9, 137, 140

Umbanda 9, 132, 133, 135, 136
United Kingdom 7, 23
universal/universality 144, 146, 151, 153–156

veil/veiling 27–29, 31–41
Vodou 124, 129

Wilson, C. Roderick 8
Winston, Sam 6, 17–25

yoga 200–202, 206–209, 218

Zeus 4, 87, 89
ziening 152, 155, 157

www.ingramcontent.com/pod-product-compliance
Lightning Source LLC
Chambersburg PA
CBHW062021220426
43662CB00010B/1422